RVUs at Work

Relative Value Units in a Changing Reimbursement World

— THIRD EDITION —

By **Max Reiboldt**, CPA
Justin Chamblee, MAcc, CPA
Coker Group

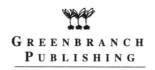

GREENBRANCH
PUBLISHING

PUBLISHER
Nancy Collins

EDITORIAL ASSISTANT
Jennifer Weiss

BOOK DESIGNER
Laura Carter
Carter Publishing Studio

COPYEDITOR
Patricia George

ABOUT THE AUTHORS

Max Reiboldt, CPA

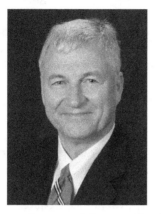

Max Reiboldt is president/CEO of Coker Group with 45 years of total experience; the last 26 years specifically focused on healthcare. He has seen first-hand the incredible changes of healthcare providers, which uniquely equips him to handle strategic, tactical, financial, and management issues that health systems and physicians face in today's evolving marketplace.

From his extensive work with health systems/hospitals, medical practices, and related healthcare entities, Mr. Reiboldt understands the nuances of the healthcare industry, especially in such a dynamic age. He understands healthcare organizations' needs to maintain viability in a highly-competitive market. His position of having "experienced everything" in the healthcare industry equips him to provide pertinent counsel to clients. Whether a transitional provider or a more cutting-edge healthcare entity, Mr. Reiboldt is particularly equipped to work with these organizations to provide sound solutions to every day and long-range challenges.

As president/CEO, Mr. Reiboldt oversees Coker Group's services and the general operations of the Firm. He has a passion for working with clients to provide sound financial, strategic, and tactical solutions to hospitals and health systems, medical practices, and other healthcare entities through keen analysis and problem-solving. Working with organizations of all sizes, Reiboldt engages in consulting projects nationwide.

An avid writer and speaker, Mr. Reiboldt enjoys educating healthcare leaders through books, white papers, articles, and speaking at national symposiums. His expertise encompasses physician/hospital alignment initiatives, hospital service line development, clinical integration initiatives, financial analyses (including physician compensation plans), mergers and acquisitions, hospital and practice strategic planning, ancillary services development, PHO/IPA/MSO/CIN development, appraisals, and "accountable care era" consultation. As the industry moves to adapt to many changes in response to healthcare reform, including the entire "volume-to-value" paradigm, he leads Coker Group's efforts in this arena.

Mr. Reiboldt is an honor graduate of Harding University with an Accounting degree.

Justin Chamblee, MAcc, CPA

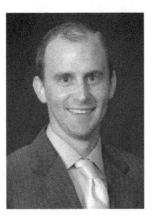

Justin Chamblee, MAcc, CPA, is a senior vice president and director of operations at Coker Group. As an executive healthcare consultant and certified public accountant, he provides strategic and financial counsel to healthcare organizations, physician practices, and healthcare attorneys throughout the country, dealing primarily with physician compensation and hospital-physician transactions. His work in physician compensation involves strategy by assisting healthcare organizations to restructure their compensation arrangements to ensure they are consistent with the market on a macro and micro basis.

Mr. Chamblee's work also involves compensation valuation by helping healthcare organizations ensure that their financial arrangements comply with the requirements of fair market value and commercial reasonableness. His other areas of expertise include contract negotiations, sale/acquisition negotiations, strategic planning and business plan development, and other areas of finance.

As a recognized thought leader, Mr. Chamblee frequently presents at national conferences where physician leaders, healthcare legal counsel, and health system administrators gather to gain knowledge in the areas of physician compensation and hospital-physician integration. He has also authored several books and professional publications in collaboration with Greenbranch Publishing, Healthcare Financial Management Association, the American Medical Association, and HealthLeaders Media.

In addition to his consulting role, Mr. Chamblee is Coker's director of operations, directing the day-to-day functioning of the company.

He has a BBA in Accounting and a Master's in Accounting from Abilene Christian University, is licensed as a Certified Public Accountant in the State of Texas, and is a member of the American Institute of Certified Public Accountants. Additionally, he has completed extensive training through the Harvard Business School Leadership program.

CONTRIBUTORS

Thomas D. Anthony, JD, Esq.

Tom Anthony, chair of Frost Brown Todd's Healthcare Industry practice, focuses on healthcare, corporate transactions, regulatory, and joint ventures. He provides advice on Stark, Anti-Kickback, and all other healthcare regulatory matters. Also, he is counsel to hospitals regarding clinically integrated networks, medical staff bylaws, physician relations, acquisition of medical groups, corporate governance, acquisitions of outpatient and ancillary facilities, strategic alliances and joint ventures, the establishment of provider-based facilities, executive employment agreements, Medicare compliance, contracting, and employment matters. Mr. Anthony also represents several senior living owners and operators in mergers/acquisitions, regulatory, patient rights, and financings.

Holding a BS from Miami University, Mr. Anthony received his JD from Case Western Reserve University School of Law.

Jeffery Daigrepont

Jeffery Daigrepont, senior vice president of Coker Group, specializes in healthcare automation, system integration, operations, and deployment of enterprise information systems for large integrated delivery networks. A popular national speaker, he is frequently engaged by highly respected organizations across the nation, including many non-profit trade associations and state medical societies.

Mr. Daigrepont authored a top-selling book, *Complete Guide and Toolkit to Successful EHR Adoption*, published by HIMSS in 2011, and was a contributing author to Coker's book, *The Healthcare Executive's Guide to ACO Strategy*, released March 2012. Mr. Daigrepont is often interviewed by various national media outlets and is frequently quoted in publications.

Mr. Daigrepont has chaired the Ambulatory Information Systems Steering Committee and has held various roles of the Healthcare Information Management Systems Society (HIMSS). He is credentialed by the American Academy of Medical Management (AAMM) with an Executive Fellowship in Practice Management (EFMP).

He also serves as an independent investment advisor to many of the nation's top healthcare venture capital firms such as Kleiner Perkins Caufield & Byers (KPCB) and Silver Lake Partners.

Aimee Greeter, MPH, FACHE

Aimee Greeter is a senior vice president at Coker Group with specialized experience in alignment, accountable care responsiveness, hospital service line development, clinical integration initiatives, strategic planning, compensation, mergers and collaborations, operational issues, and financial management. Ms. Greeter works with non-profit and for-profit hospitals and health systems of all sizes, and larger single and multi-specialty physician practices to achieve their strategic and tactical goals.

As the co-leader of Coker's Finance, Operations, and Strategy (FOS) group, Ms. Greeter manages the firm's financial and transaction services for healthcare facilities throughout the country. The team of more than ten consultants works with some of the largest and most prestigious health systems in the U.S., as well as regional health systems, medical centers, critical access hospitals, outpatient facilities, and medical practices in all 50 states. Additionally, the FOS team regularly works with major for-profit healthcare entities on their financial and transaction strategies, including assisting on buy-side acquisitions, divestiture of assets, and strategic development plans.

A popular program speaker, Ms. Greeter is frequently engaged by highly respected organizations across the nation to speak to health systems, medical groups, legal associations, and other healthcare constituents. Her accomplishments include the authorship of numerous articles and books, and Ms. Greeter often gives interviews and is noted in healthcare industry publications.

Ms. Greeter attained a BS in Human Biology with honors from Michigan State University, and an MPH in Health Policy and Management from the Rollins School of Public Health at Emory University.

Jeff Gorke

Jeff Gorke brings approximately 27 years of healthcare experience to the position of senior vice president with Coker Group. His primary focus is on strategic and operational work assisting clients in macro- and microstructural change to enhance processes and programs, drive efficiencies, and improve profitability. He uses his experience to help clients with operational assessments, physician compensation reviews, employed physician network turnarounds, financial and revenue cycle assessments, and strategic planning.

Mr. Gorke has a record of designing, operationalizing, and implementing strategic initiatives to improve overall performance for clients helping them prepare for impending shifts in care delivery and reimbursement models. Specifically, he manages strategic and operational components concurrently to improve planning, governance, and top-line management while assuring operational sustainability by driving programs from efficient day-to-day management to billing/collections and data mining for physician groups and healthcare systems. Mr. Gorke has also led in the selection and implementation of electronic medical records systems (EMRs) and utilized data mining for clinical efficiency and financial modeling. He quantifies his engagements empowering clients to measure their outcomes and gauge their ROIs while managing their projects.

Mr. Gorke holds a BBA from Temple University and an MBA from the University of Richmond.

Ellis M. ("Mac") Knight, MD

Mac Knight is senior vice president and chief medical officer of Coker Group. With over 30 years in the healthcare arena, he has attained significant experience and knowledge in this industry.

Before joining Coker, Dr. Knight served in several executive roles for Palmetto Health in Columbia, South Carolina. There, he oversaw Palmetto Health's employed physician network, ambulatory services division (rehab, lab, home health, hospice care, and imaging), and helped to develop and manage their clinical integration program. Earlier, he was Palmetto Health Richland's vice president for medical affairs.

Dr. Knight graduated from Stanford University with a BA in Human Biology and received his doctor of medicine degree, cum laude, from the University of Oregon Health Science Center's School of Medicine. He earned an MBA from the University of Massachusetts at Amherst. He holds fellowships in the American College of Physicians, the Society of Hospital Medicine, and the American College of Healthcare Executives.

Dr. Knight oversees Coker Group's hospital strategy and operations services and is Coker Group's chief medical officer. He has particular expertise in population health management, clinical care process design, cost accounting, hospital revenue cycle management, and hospital-physician integration. He is familiar with the management and operations of rural hospitals, community hospitals, public hospitals, and large health system to include academic medical centers.

Mark Reiboldt, MSc

Mark Reiboldt is a senior vice president and director of strategy at Coker Group, where he specializes in financial advisory and transaction services for hospitals, health systems, and other healthcare organizations. These transactions include mergers and acquisitions, divestitures, equity purchases, physician alignment deals, and joint ventures. His advisory services often entail acquisition/investment due diligence, valuation services, transaction management, buy-side representation, strategic alternatives processes, and post-merger integration.

Mr. Reiboldt regularly presents at numerous national and regional conferences on a variety of topics, such as healthcare financial transactions, valuation trends, capital markets issues, and healthcare public policy. He has also contributed as an author on articles and books for a variety of publications covering a wide range of topics related to his area of focus, and his pieces are featured in numerous industry and mainstream media publications.

Mr. Reiboldt received an MSc in financial economics from the University of London and a BA in political science from Georgia State University. He also completed the High Potentials Leadership executive management program at Harvard Business School. Mark is a member of the board of directors of the Coker Foundation, which oversees healthcare and aid relief initiatives in the U. S. and abroad.

ACKNOWLEDGEMENTS

As the editor, I would like to thank the contributors to this edition. Their level of proficiency continues to impress me. Each chapter represents the know-how derived from many years of hands-on work with clients and in-depth knowledge of the subject matter. Also, Coker Group expressly appreciates the contribution by Thomas Anthony, Esq., of Frost Brown Todd, for his expertise in healthcare law.

Lastly, we thank Greenbranch Publishing and Nancy Collins. We appreciate our continuing working relationship with the entire Greenbranch team. Thank you for your confidence.

Kay B. Stanley, FACMPE, Editor

TABLE OF CONTENTS

PREFACE

RVUs at Work: Value Units in a Changing Reimbursement World is the third edition in a series originally published in 2010 and followed by the release of the second edition in 2014. The fast-paced transition in the healthcare industry's reimbursement mechanisms can confuse and overwhelm providers without a foundation to gain perspective. This edition intends to lay the groundwork, differentiate the past and present, and sort through what reimbursement methods are pending in some areas of the country and what is occurring in more progressive regions.

Chapter 1 recaps the recent history and background of units of measurement. It addresses the evolution of RVUs and introduces other units of measurement. Next is the discussion of how RVUs will factor in a value-based reimbursement era and the anticipated changes that are apt to occur.

Chapter 2 presents MACRA and Units of Measurement. Topics include developing MIPS and APMs and reimbursing physicians under MACRA reimbursement.

Chapter 3 addresses physician-hospital alignment in a value-based environment. Discussion encompasses the alignment market and specific alignment tools. It emphasizes the importance of educating physicians on the new environment and concludes with the presentation of RVUs within alignment models.

Chapter 4 is the chapter on compensation in a value-based reimbursement world. Both private practice and hospital-employed settings are the focus of the information, including the long-term expectations for using RVUs. Also covered are arrangements for RVUs and quality incentives.

In Chapter 5, a prominent healthcare attorney considers legal issues of the value-based reimbursement era encompassing the anticipated changes, fair market value, and commercially reasonable parameters in conjunction with MACRA regulations.

The playbook for wRVU-based alignment structures and alignment models is the subject matter of Chapter 6. Discussion includes the relevance of productivity units, practice management applications, and quality units' applications.

Chapter 7 explores value units and technology, opening with an overview of the current healthcare landscape relative to technology and value-based reimbursement, and extending with software and care coordination.

Management in a hybrid reimbursement environment performance measurement is explored in Chapter 8, encompassing analytics, accountability, strategic planning, and tactical considerations.

Chapter 9 lays out care process design, value-based units and care coordination, and management efficiency and care coordination. This chapter also describes revenue cycle functions and the role of RVUs in care of coordination.

The final chapter, Chapter 10, expounds on RVUs and the future, new forms of value units, educating and acclimating providers, strategic planning within the new reimbursement realm, and concludes with value units and clinical integration.

Together, the chapters unwrap the critical issues in the transition from a fee-for-service to a fee-for-value-based payment system and present solutions for handling these challenges. The essential matters are to ensure that providers get paid for all the services they render and to secure the right technology to attain the necessary data.

Readers will gain a level of competency in an otherwise confusing reimbursement system.

CHAPTER 1

Recent History and Background of Units of Measurement

In light of the move toward value-based reimbursement and the trajectory from volume-to-value, some would argue that relative value units (RVUs) and other units of measurement of productivity will soon be outdated, even obsolete. However, regardless of the reimbursement paradigm and variations that result from productivity-based reimbursement, health systems, physicians, and related individuals who provide healthcare will be compelled to monitor, track, and measure productivity.

Historically, productivity has been measured in various ways, including gross and net charges, gross and net collections, patient encounters, or the number of procedures within a healthcare provider's purview. These types of productivity measures allow for inconsistencies. Further, even the definitions vary in some instances.

When RVUs were introduced, they quickly became the prevailing system for measuring and monitoring physician and related provider productivity, transcending to a reliable basis for determining reimbursement and, later, compensation. The mere presence of current procedural terminology (CPT) codes and their relationship with units of production and RVUs continue to be the most consistent and fair way of measuring productivity.

RVUS AT A GLANCE

RVUs are made up of three components: work, practice expense, and malpractice. By far, the most prominent of the three is work-only RVUs (wRVUs); they represent just over 50% of the total RVU value. The practice expense component (overhead) is worth about 44%, with malpractice at 4% percent. These percentages make up a single RVU unit.

Traditionally, RVUs (mainly, wRVUs) are converted to a compensation total via the conversion factor. This formula also applies to the reimbursement structure, though it is applied to the total RVU. The Centers for Medicare and Medicaid Services (CMS) has continued to use this methodology with some variations, such as the geographic adjustment factor or geographic cost indices. These elements adjust for cost differences based on geographical locations and also consider cost of living and social, economic, and environmental factors. The geographical practice cost indices are multiplied by each RVU component and then added to obtain the total RVU value.

Thus, RVUs continue to function as a viable form of reimbursement methodology in calculations and are relevant to all areas of evaluation of performance by governmental payers and private payers alike.

RVUS AND EVOLVING MEASUREMENT

The use of RVUs began in the late 1980s and early 1990s. Their history has been one of consistent development, and today they serve as a significant part of every medical practice's evaluation of performance and reimbursement. Beginning with the American Medical Association's (AMA) relative value scale, RVUs have continued to be a fundamental way to measure productivity.

The relative value scale update committee (RUC) was created in 1991 to act as an advisory group to CMS and has served as a means to update RVU values by CPT code every five years. CMS has accepted most of the RUC's recommendations for many years.

Medicare has utilized a conversion factor to derive total reimbursement notwithstanding the geographical adjustments as outlined above. Thus, RVUs have continued to evolve as the most prominent means of measuring productivity. In a value-based reimbursement system, they most likely will continue to serve as a major area of productivity measurement and reimbursement determination. (Note: We believe that even in an evolving value-based reimbursement system, volume-based payments will continue to prevail for some time and may always be the most prominent means of reimbursement.)

Thus, the uses of RVUs today are myriad, including as a:

- Means to determine reimbursement;
- Means to measure and evaluate provider productivity;
- Means to measure cost;
- Benchmarking standard for surveys;
- Determinate of provider compensation; and
- Basis (or foundation) for negotiating contract rates with payers.

Will each of these uses of RVUs continue in a value-based system? We believe that most or all will remain; therefore, it is important to continue to learn more about RVUs and to apply them to the day-to-day management of medical practices.

RVUs likely will continue to evolve as the industry shifts toward value-based reimbursement. Due to their flexibility and their capacity to level the playing ground, they will continue to be applicable and significant. For example, as bundled payments become a part of the value-based reimbursement structure, RVUs should help to determine how those bundled payments are allocated among the various providers. What better means is there to complete such allocations than via RVUs among those providers that generate professional fees?

It is important to note that RVUs probably will continue to have a place in our evaluation process, and value-based reimbursement will not impugn their use. Nevertheless, other forms of productivity measurement, including various units of measurement, may be considered increasingly in the future.

OTHER UNITS OF MEASUREMENT

Over time, while RVUs continue to be the predominate units of measurement, other types of measurements have evolved over the years. Let's take a brief look at some examples.

Time RVUs

An alternative to the traditional RVU measurement is measuring value (or unit of productivity) based on the time spent delivering the service. Depending on the interest and actual utilization, time RVUs may be most applicable or even a fair method of assessment in some settings, such as when processes take more time, even though they may be awarded fewer RVUs under the standard system of measurement—such as dental procedures. The use of this methodology is especially pertinent to specialties like cardiology.

While time RVUs are not a standardized system, they may increase in prominence, as value-based reimbursement is becoming more the norm. In other words, if the time that is involved in completing a procedure or a particular encounter is more relevant (and particularly more pertinent to the value-based reimbursement structure), such units of productivity may likewise be more applicable than the standard RVU system.

Assignment of Qualitative or Non-Procedural Work and RVUs

The assignment of qualitative or non-procedural work structure awards RVUs for services not directly tied to a CPT code. We have always used these (somewhat arbitrarily) and without substantial standardization. However, when consistently applied within each setting, they may be applicable.

Activities that consume a provider's time and do not necessarily contribute directly to a patient care revenue yet are still valuable to the overall service offering often fit this metric. Factors such as serving the community, performing leadership or administrative duties, as well as quality clinical outcomes, patient satisfaction, and effectively controlling cost are all a part of such qualitative RVUs.

Although these measures are often subjective, with more standardization within the value-based reimbursement settings, these forms of productivity may well have a greater emphasis.

Total Cost of Care and Resource Use Measurement

In 2012, the U. S. National Quality Forum endorsed the total cost of care and resource use (TCOC) measure developed by HealthPartners in Minnesota (2017).[1]

This measure essentially equates to total cost as being equal to resource use times price.

TCOC uses total cost relative resource value (TCRRV), which are units designed to evaluate resource use across all types of medical services, procedures, and places of service and facilitate the comparison of them. TCRRVs are based on weighing Medicare Severity-Diagnosis Related Groups (MS-DRGs), RVUs, and ambulatory payment classifications. They are calibrated to reflect a uniform resource value for services that require similar resources regardless where they are performed, such as a laboratory or even in a physician's office performing EEGs, etc.

These types of measurements can be used to evaluate providers, hospitals, and health plans against their peers on their efficiency of resource use in treating similar conditions and overall care of a population. This form of reimbursement is pertinent in a value-based setting. In fact, these metrics form the essence of such a unit of measurement process evaluation.

Thus, while RVUs in the traditional sense will continue to be a significant part of performance measurement, even in a value-based structure, some of these newer forms of measurement units will become more applicable in a value-based setting.

RVUS IN A VALUE-BASED REIMBURSEMENT ERA

After considering the above variables and continuing to highlight the importance of RVUs in a value-based reimbursement structure, there are some key points to consider.

While value-based reimbursement encourages healthcare providers to deliver the best care at the lowest cost, RVUs and measurements of productivity (even those other units of measurements discussed in the previous paragraphs) will continue to be a necessary component of the overall process and evaluation. Under the value-based system, providers should focus on care management, reducing cost, collecting and utilizing data, and overall population health management. This will be done in various manners and through various mediums or vehicles. Clinically integrated networks (CINs), accountable care organizations (ACOs), medical home and the like will all be a part of this process.

Value-based reimbursement programs will include specific forms of payment tied to procedural and surgical bundles, pay for performance, and shared savings plans. Inevitably, the measurement of productivity will still be relevant, and RVUs should be accumulated, even though they may not have quite the impact on reimbursement that they do today.

Another factor to consider is how fast we will move to value-based reimbursement. RVUs may still be the predominant methodology for measuring productivity and reimbursement and provider compensation, even into the next 5 to 10 years. Why? The reason may well lie in the fact that value-based reimbursement, while being spoken about and logical, may not materialize from both the government and the commercial payer marketplace. Simply stated, if the payers do not actively and more aggressively move to value-based reimbursement, it just will not exist, and RVUs may return to the level or predominance that they hold today and have held for the past 15 to 20 years or more.

While RVUs were not designed to incorporate considerations of quality of care or patient outcomes, features that are essential in a value-based reimbursement structure, the need to measure productivity will continue for the reasons we've presented. And even with the introduction of the Medicare Access and CHIP Reauthorization Act (MACRA) and the Merit Incentive Payment System (MIPS) or alternative payment models, productivity in measurements of RVUs likely still will be a major part of this entire reimbursement process. For example, MIPS measures and payment rates based on a composite score are considering the following percentages:

- Quality—50%
- Advancing care information—25%
- Clinical improvement—15%
- Resource use—10%

While none of these measures are directly related to productivity, the overall government reimbursement to healthcare providers within the MACRA legislation is much less than for fee-for-service reimbursement. That is, even with the MACRA regulation requirements, government reimbursement will still lean significantly toward fee-for-service.

Though RVUs are expected to be in use for the foreseeable future, there may be adjustments to their structure or use. Possibilities may include incorporating a quality- or performance-based component to the total RVU. We discuss this issue further in later chapters of this book, but it would be perfectly logical to add to the RVU components a quality metric, not unlike the three that currently exist (i.e., work, practice expense, and malpractice expense).

Another consideration would be shifting the use of RVUs more to performance evaluation measures or efficiency measures, based on cost per RVU. Again, this fits the value-based model well as we will explore later in this book.

Another example of changes anticipated is using RVUs to determine the most efficient allocation of resources under bundled payment models. This could entail a new breakthrough in the utilization and importance of RVUs in a value-based reimbursement paradigm.

Finally, the changing RVU utilization could be that we recognize new and current Medicare payment CPT codes for non-face-to-face or prolonged evaluation of management services and increase the RVU values, and, thus, the payment rates for such services. Telemedicine, for example, is becoming a prominent non-face-to-face provider strategy.

As technology continues to improve, the ability for physicians and other providers to have appropriate and effective contact with the patient yet not in the same room, face-to-face, is likely. This arrangement will help to account for the types of services and time spent in value-based services, such as coordinating care, providing education to the patient and local caregiver, and working toward wellness and prevention activities.

While strictly speaking, we may be considering value-based reimbursement, applying these types of metrics and expanding definitions of RVU values (such as a quality RVU component) will continue to result in the applicability of RVUs.

CONCLUSION

RVUs, over time, have proved to be a most useful source for measuring productivity. It is universally accepted as the standard for measuring physician and related provider productivity. RVUs serve as the basis for determining reimbursement and compensation, plus appropriate cost indicators. As we move to a value-based reimbursement structure, the question of the viability and usefulness of RVUs is valid.

In this chapter, we have reviewed several areas that will enhance the utilization of RVUs within a value-based system, which likely will remain as mostly a fee-for-service environment, at least for the foreseeable future. As a result, collecting performance data based on RVUs will become increasingly important, not only in continuing to capture and analyze productivity, but also in using these data as at least a portion of the basis for measuring quality and clinical outcomes and related distribution formulas.

Exactly how RVUs will be used in new systems, starting with the MACRA legislation as it is enacted, plus as ACOs and CINs continue to develop, is a question we will consider and provide insights on in subsequent chapters of this book.

Flexibility in the utilization of RVUs under this new structure—however it develops—will be necessary. New forms of unit productivity measurements may be introduced, even to the extent of including a quality component within the standard RVU derivation. In other words, what has always been a three-component RVU (work, practice expense, and malpractice premiums) may have a fourth added tied strictly to quality. That indicator will be determined based on the overall performance and outcomes of the practitioner.

Continuing through the chapters of this book, we will consider areas of applicability relative to RVUs and value-based reimbursement. We will discuss many areas of application from physician/hospital alignment in a value-based environment to considerations of compensation in such a structure to legal matters. Yes, we will also discuss MACRA and how it may affect RVUs and their utilization.

In later chapters, we will consider examples of both cost and unit productivity applications, value units, technology, and ultimately, the overall consideration of how a hybrid reimbursement environment will be affected by various units of measurement, including RVUs.

Our overarching conclusion is that RVUs will continue to be relevant in our healthcare delivery system and the measurements of productivity and overall performance of physicians and related providers.

REFERENCE

1. HealthPartners. *Total cost of care (TCOC) and total resource use*. HealthPartners. September 21, 2017. https://www.healthpartners.com/ucm/groups/public/@hp/@public/documents/documents/dev_057649.pdf. Accessed August 28, 2017.

CHAPTER 2

MACRA and Units of Measurement

In April 2015, Congress passed with overwhelming bipartisan support the Medicare Access and CHIP Reauthorization Act, otherwise known as MACRA. This landmark piece of legislation will dramatically change the way doctors and other U. S. healthcare providers are paid by the largest payer in the country: The Centers for Medicare and Medicaid Services (CMS).

MACRA was designed to replace the sustainable growth rate (SGR) formula that Medicare had been using prior to 2015 to adjust provider payments in an attempt to slow the rate of inflation in the healthcare economy. The SGR was extremely unpopular. Once or twice a year, providers would lobby hard for Congress to pass a "doc-fix" bill that would relieve them of perceived draconian cuts in CMS reimbursement rates. Finally, in early 2015, the Congress not only repealed the SGR but replaced it with MACRA, a much different piece of legislation.

In brief, MACRA and its quality payment programs (QPPs) will move CMS from primarily a fee-for-service payment model to a fee-for-value payment model. Here, providers' reimbursements depend on the provision of services and how well those services were rendered across four basic categories of performance.

MACRA's performance metrics are broken down into the following basic categories:

1. **Quality.** Standard measures of quality, e.g., those included in the Healthcare Effectiveness Data and Information Set (HEDIS) developed by the National Clinical Quality Association or NCQA, are used to gauge provider performance across all specialties and locations of clinical care delivery, inpatient, outpatient, community, virtual, etc. This data can be submitted directly by providers to CMS via the CMS website; it can be uploaded to CMS through clinical data registries; or, it can be transmitted via certain electronic health record (EHR) systems that are capable of both collecting and reporting such information.

2. **Cost.** These include measures of cost to CMS and compare provider's practice efficiencies with peer groups of Medicare providers across the country. This data is retrieved from claims data submitted to CMS for payment by Medicare and Medicaid providers of all types.

3. **Clinical Practice Improvement Activities (CPIA).** A new category of performance developed specifically by CMS for the MACRA QPPs, providers are asked to implement quality or care improvement activities designed to improve

health equity, behavioral and mental health, beneficiary engagement, care coordination, emergency response and preparedness, expanded practice access, patient safety and practice assessment, and population management. There are 92 such activities available, and the purpose is to drive performance and process improvements across all types of CMS provider organizations. These activities can also be reported in a variety of ways, through the CMS website, via a qualified clinical data registry, or via particular types of EHRs.

4. **Advancing Care Information.** This category is an expansion of CMS's meaningful use program and is geared to drive the use of electronic medical records throughout the industry. The criteria range from the ability to share records between providers to the capacity to submit data electronically to public health entities regarding syndromic surveillance and other issues. Performance data in this category can be submitted in several similar ways to those used for quality and CPIA activities.

In January 2019, CMS providers will have their fee-for-service reimbursement rates adjusted depending on their composite performance scores across the above four categories. These adjustments will depend on performance data collected during the calendar year 2017, i.e., the adjusted payments will be based on a two-year review of performance data. The aggregate performance scores will be calculated by combining the weighted scores for each category. Further, the quality and cost metrics will be risk adjusted using CMS's risk adjustment methodology now being used in Medicare Advantage programs to account for differences in clinical complexity, severity of illness, demographics, income level, and prevalence of chronic conditions within any one provider's patient population.

It is important to know that the quality and cost categories of MACRA performance measures will be risk adjusted using CMS's Hierarchical Condition Category or HCC risk adjustment methodology. This measurement involves capturing information regarding an individual patient's clinical conditions from the medical record, assigning each condition to its appropriate ICD-10 diagnostic code, and then categorizing these codes into what are known as hierarchical clinical conditions.

There are currently just over 100 HCCs that classify the over 9,000 ICD-10 codes. Each HCC is weighted as to the risk it conveys to the patient to whom it is assigned. These risk weightings are combined with other features of a provider's patient population (in this case of MACRA, Medicare beneficiaries) such as gender, age, disability, income level, and other demographic factors that affect risk. The final risk adjustment factor (RAF) score then determines how a provider's performance measures are adjusted to account for the clinical complexity, severity of illness, and other risks inherent in their patient pool.

This risk adjustment methodology will require that Medicare providers pay greater attention than ever before to clinical documentation, especially in the ambulatory arena, as only appropriately documented HCCs can be captured and used for risk adjustment purposes. Providers who ignore this requirement, therefore, risk having their performance adjusted inaccurately to account for the baseline risk status of their patient population and subsequently not receiving the credit they deserve for effectively and efficiently managing their Medicare patients.

MIPS OR APMS

The two QPPs that are prescribed by the MACRA legislation encompass the Merit Incentive Payment System (MIPS) wherein individual providers or groups are evaluated regarding their performance within the four categories outlined below and the alternative payment models (APMs) which include innovative provider organizations. These include accountable care organizations (ACOs) and medical homes in which Medicare providers are eligible for a 5% increase in payments from 2019 through 2024 that replaces MIPS adjustments to compensation and rewards participation in one of the advanced APMs. It is clear that CMS, over time, would like all providers to participate in APMs; however, currently, the number of these alternatives to MIPS are limited. More advanced APMs that qualify for the 5% bonus increases will likely be rolled out over time, and providers can look forward to having more options available to gain exemption from MIPS.

Providers and provider groups who are trying to determine in which payment model they should operate under MACRA need to consider the following questions:

1. *With which type of risk are they most comfortable?* It is important to remember that both MIPS and APMs put a component of provider compensation at risk for performance. Under the MIPS model, the risk entails performing against the metrics within the four categories of performance outlined above. Under APMs, the risk may seem to be less since the 5% bonus for participating in an APM is not dependent on performance. Nevertheless, APM participants' performance across the four MACRA categories will be measured, and the participants' performance scores will determine their rewards or liabilities within any particular APM.

   For example, participants in a Medicare Shared Savings Program ACO will receive a share of the savings or have to pay back a percentage of the loss depending on the overall ability of the ACO to cut costs. Moreover, it is likely that provider performance scores will determine the proportion of the savings or loss each provider will be eligible to receive or be liable for paying. Ultimately, providers need to consider their capabilities to drive performance across all four MACRA performance categories and determine the capability of any particular APM to achieve their goals (cost savings, quality improvement, etc.) when deciding which type of program to enter. Only with close scrutiny can they determine whether they would be at more or less risk in MIPS or any specific APM.

2. *Are they eligible for available advanced APMs?* As noted, very few APM options are currently available. Most providers during the first few years of MACRA's roll out will be in MIPS. Over time, the number of advanced APMs available will increase. Some will be very specialty-specific, e.g., oncology medical homes and end-stage renal disease programs, which will be relevant to practitioners in these areas. Therefore, all providers should look for APMs that meet their needs and strongly consider moving from MIPS to an APM when possible.

3. *Are there economies of scale and group purchasing advantages to joining an APM?* The reporting requirements and IT infrastructure needs of MACRA participation may be more than individual providers or small groups can afford on their own. APMs allow multiple providers to band together and share operating costs under this reimbursement model. Additionally, APMs are likely to have staff to whom small practices can off-load some of the more time-intensive elements of MACRA participation, such as data aggregation and reporting.

4. *Which option will be more likely to benefit your practice as to pay for performance increases?* If your perspective is that you or your group is a top performer, you may not want to have your performance measures diluted by co-mingling them with others in an APM. On the other hand, if you're not confident of your performance level, you may want to band with others who can help you attain higher performance levels and higher levels of rewards.

ALIGNING REIMBURSEMENT AND COMPENSATION

As it relates to provider compensation models, MACRA likely will be the source of many non-production, performance-based metrics used to create hybrid production/performance-based compensation plans. This type of plan will become more common as value-based reimbursements, such as MACRA, are introduced and employers of physicians and other healthcare providers attempt to align reimbursements with compensation.

To demonstrate, consider a hospital-owned internal medicine practice where the average physician currently receives total compensation of $200,000 per a work relative value unit (wRVU) productivity-based compensation model. Should the hospital want to align its compensation plan more closely with one of their major payers, i.e., CMS (Medicare), it could do this by selecting several of the proposed MACRA quality, clinical practice improvement, cost, or advancing care information measures to use as incentive targets for the individual physicians.

Next, the hospital might choose to place 10%, or $20,000, of each physician's total compensation at risk for achieving these incentive goals. The targeted goals and the amount of incentive around each goal might look like Figure 2.1.

Note in the hypothetical example illustrated in Figure 2.1: the goal categories match up with the performance categories in MACRA. Again, this should serve the organization to align and engage their front-line providers/physicians toward efforts that will result in higher reimbursements from Medicare through either of MACRA's QPP models.

Next, note that the thresholds for goal achievement in this model are all set using an "all-or-nothing" payout model. This will make the incentive model easy to administer and avoid confusion when calculating performance bonuses.

Be aware that the amount moved from productivity-based compensation to performance-based compensation is small relative to the entire physician compensation package (10%). While performance or value-based reimbursement (VBR) models seem to be the wave of the future, these VBRs are unlikely to replace more traditional fee-for-service-based reimbursement plans altogether.

	FIGURE 2.1. Targeted Goals and Incentives			
Goal Category	**Goal specifics**	**Goal Achieved Y/N**	**$$ At Risk**	**$$ Paid**
Quality	90% or more of diabetic patients have a hemoglobin A1c level of less than 8	Y	$2,000.00	$2,000.00
Quality	90% of hypertensive patients have an average blood pressure of less than 140/90	N	$2,000.00	$0.00
Clinical Practice Improvement Activity	Two CPIAs performed within the practice over the last year	N	$2,000.00	$0.00
Advancing Care Information	Practice can transmit and receive medication lists via EMR	Y	$2,000.00	$2,000.00
Cost Control	Medicare average patient costs less than benchmark average	Y	$2,000.00	$2,000.00
			TOTAL	$6,000.00

Further compensation formulations can be used to combine wRVUs with performance measures to determine provider payments. For instance, the dollar per wRVU rate paid to any one provider can be adjusted up or down to incorporate quality and other non-productivity performance measures. As an example, see Figure 2.2.

FIGURE 2.2. Example of Compensation Formulations		
Performance Goals Achieved	**Dollar per wRVU Payment Rate**	**Additional Pay for Provider Producing 10,000 wRVUs / Year**
$0.00	$50.00	$0.00
$1.00	$52.00	$2,000.00
$2.00	$54.00	$4,000.00
$3.00	$56.00	$6,000.00
$4.00	$58.00	$8,000.00
$5.00	$60.00	$10,000.00

In the example, a physician producing 10,000 wRVUs a year and receiving payment of $50 per wRVU would receive an increase in his or her dollar per wRVU rate, depending on how they performed against five performance measures. Achieving each performance measure would increase the physician's wRVU payment rate by two dollars ($2,000 overall) and up to $10,000 in performance bonus incentive payments could be paid to this provider to incentivize performance against these goals.

CONCLUSION

MACRA will require those who operate under its often arcane and confusing rules to master an understanding of the way this transformative payment plan measures provider performance and uses those metrics to determine payments for services. These criteria will be especially challenging in an era when the measurement of quality in the healthcare system is still a nascent science, and measurement of other parameters, such as cost, has not been a priority for most providers.

Accurate data capture, aggregation, and reporting of quality measures and deployment of true cost accounting systems will require IT systems with capabilities provided by few, if any, healthcare IT vendors at this time. Indeed, this payment model will also require a transformation across the industry of the basic business model that underpins the healthcare delivery system. This much change will not come easily, and the transformation is unlikely to be smooth. Nevertheless, the tipping point appears to have been reached, and MACRA is likely to be the first of many large-scale, value-based, population health payment plans with many more yet to come.

Providers, therefore, should avail themselves of all possible information about the standards by which they will be evaluated as the shift from volume to value in the healthcare economy inexorably proceeds. Those subject to this dramatic sea change in the reimbursement system should also learn how to retool the delivery system to ensure that their measures of performance continue to improve and more reliable, safe, and efficient care is provided to the patients served. Mechanisms for doing this will be covered in more detail in Chapter 9 of this book. Suffice it to say for now that this re-tooling of the delivery system will also not be easy, smooth, or swift. Medical science will need to concern itself with activities, such as population health management, once thought outside the realm of our traditional care delivery system.

As is often stated, you cannot change what you do not measure. The performance metrics for MACRA that will likely also be used as incentive goals for third-generation compensation plans are just that: measures. What is more important than how we measure quality, costs, and other parameters of performance, is how we go about improving our performance in these areas and whether these performance improvement processes are data-driven. In other words, the key to understanding MACRA performance measures is to make sure they are the basis for understanding performance and driving that performance forward and improving care delivery so that it delivers higher value to the healthcare consumer.

CHAPTER 3

Physician-Hospital Alignment in a Value-Based Environment

Working together, faster, smarter, harder— the term "working" is used in many ways, which is a clear sign of the emphasis we place on "working" in today's culture. In healthcare, "working together" may be the most representative description of the recipe for success as we transition more fully into the value-based reimbursement era.

The developing emphasis on quality and cost requires physicians and hospitals to come together and work collaboratively to meet their respective goals. In this chapter, we examine both the strategic and structural considerations of alignment, integration, and engagement in the midst of today's changing healthcare environment.

OVERVIEW OF ALIGNMENT MARKET

During the past seven years, there has been a steady push toward alignment in the healthcare industry. This focus on alignment has fostered consolidation, created critical mass, and impacted market shares, all of which are the *historical* goals of alignment. However, in today's environment, the goals of alignment are not, and should not be, the same as they have been in the past. Instead, alignment must now focus on aligning the parties' incentives.

Earlier alignment models rewarded production (both in the physicians' compensation plans, which were often based on wRVU generation, and in the hospital's greater revenue from higher volume). In contrast, contemporary alignment must focus on both the numerator and denominator of the value equation (that being outcomes and cost, respectively). Therefore, current alignment plans must move beyond production-only and consider the ways physicians and hospitals can genuinely increase quality and bend the cost curve, and do so in a collaborative fashion.

As a result, the hallmarks of previous alignment transactions are changing as the value-based environment takes hold. For the next five years, we will see the transition from structural alignment-only to an alignment that is building toward integration. While alignment is still essential, as it is the primary framework of the physician/hospital relationship, the incentives and tenor of these physician/hospital relationships will change from structural-only to strategic as well.

The focus of integration will be gaining efficiencies and reducing costs, true collaboration and sharing of best practices, improving quality and enhancing the patient experience. While alignment establishes the hospital-physician ties necessary for group-wide, value-centric initiatives, it is clinical integration that takes it a step further and begins to tie behaviors and rewards to mutual goals more holistically. (See Figure 3.1 for the connectedness behind these concepts.) So, why are both clinical and operational integration necessary? A few notable reasons include the following factors:

- MACRA (MIPS/APMs)
- Shared savings
- Bundled payments
- Patient-Centered Medical Home
- Value-based incentives
- Capitation

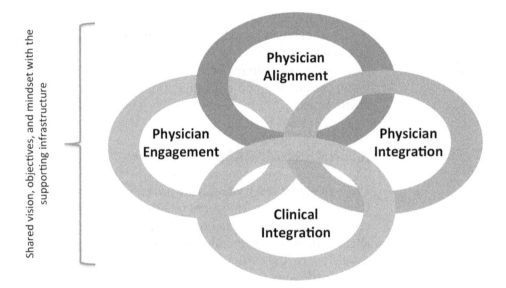

FIGURE 3.1. Alignment, Engagement, and Integration as Primary Drivers for Increasing Value

These legislative and reimbursement realities are beginning to drive physician and hospital behaviors. As the saying goes, "money talks." Because both commercial and governmental payers are changing the way providers are paid through programs like MIPS and bundled payments, there is a greater need—and incentive—for clinical and operational integration. In reality, the concept of integration has gone from being a "nice-to-have" to a strategic and operational imperative.

In summary, be aware that:

- Alignment is more often becoming the predecessor to clinical integration.
- The provision of high-quality care at lower costs must be an expectation in contemporary alignment models.
- Clinical integration between providers is a necessary precursor to value-based contracting.
- Hospitals and physicians must also have aligned incentives if they are going to contract together.
- Success within at-risk contracting must be a part of the parties' mutual goals.

SPECIFIC ALIGNMENT TOOLS

Effectuating the fundamental changes that will create the movement toward value must begin with the providers: hospitals *and* physicians. Thankfully, within the proverbial "toolbox" available to physicians and hospitals are many methods to support this movement. As noted, while integration has changed regarding its relative importance, so also has alignment as the basis for future integration efforts become increasingly necessary and more nimble. In fact, traditional alignment models are starting to morph, thus providing more alignment tools than have previously existed. For example, consider the following resources:

- *Professional Services Agreement (PSA) models* now include "carve-out" structures that feature only a portion of the practice or a specific set of services.
- *Employment models* have begun to allow physicians more autonomy than ever before.
- *ACOs/CINs* are gaining prevalence and function as an alternative to standard employment.
- *Joint equity ventures* are becoming more common.

A PSA model that has grown in popularity over the past several years is the Carve-Out PSA, which is a variant of conventional PSAs such as the Traditional PSA and the Global Payment PSA. The Carve-Out PSA involves a subset of the practice aligning with a hospital partner. A prime example is when a single specialty within a private multi-specialty practice aligns with a hospital.

This model began in earnest for cardiology after the significant cuts in their reimbursement for echo and nuclear studies in 2009. At that time, many cardiologists started looking for stability, but were reticent to leave their private practice model and become employed. As a result, many practices approached hospitals about carving out their cardiologists and forming a PSA with only those physicians from within the practice; thus, the popularity of the Carve-Out PSA began.

With its evolution, we now see this model occurring for even subspecialized physicians within a single specialty (for example, only the hand surgeons within an orthopedic practice). While the Carve-Out can take the form of any other PSA (i.e., the Traditional or Global Payment PSA), it is most often structured as a Global Payment PSA, with the overhead reimbursement limited to the direct overhead (and some limited allocated overhead) for the attributable physicians within the PSA. The reason for this new structure is that these Carve-Out PSAs allow focused contracting on a specific set of services. This narrow focus then drives limited alignment (in terms of scope) and forces constituents to work closely together on a finite list of objectives.

Unlike broader PSAs in which the drivers and incentives may spread across numerous services or even specialties, a Carve-Out PSA allows specific goals to be set and incentives distributed based on performance in comparison to only those specific goals.

Employment models have also begun to change to address the movement toward value-based contracting. For example, many more employed physician networks are contracting as an ACO or clinically integrated network (CIN) and then placing physician compensation at risk based on group performance within that ACO/CIN.

This shift is a monumental one from previous employment models where compensation was almost exclusively determined by individual performance. The concept that a group mindset could exist and compensation could be tied to that, even in employment, is truly novel. Beyond that, that the group's success would be based upon *value*, rather than *productivity*, is even more extreme! However, it is this type of novel thinking that is necessary as the entire reimbursement paradigm changes.

Some argue that the Department of Health and Human Services' (DHHS) 2015 announcement regarding value-based payments was novel, and as such, reacting to that pronouncement and others, both impacting the governmental and commercial payers, requires equally novel strategies to adapt and ultimately to be successful. We are now starting to see this ingenuity take root even in employment, perhaps the oldest form of alignment.

The one caution to these contemporary alignment models is always the legal ramifications. Hospitals must ensure that their agreements with physicians do not break Stark Law through referrals of patients. While fair market value (FMV) assessments play a significant role in ensuring this compliance, there are other nuances of the law that must be observed.

In addition to Stark Law, hospitals are also bound by federal Anti-Kickback Statutes. Relationships (PSA, employment, joint venture, etc.) must be arranged in such a way as to eliminate kickbacks from referrals of Medicare and Medicaid patients to the hospital. Although these two points cover most federal regulatory issues, a hospital also must adhere to their state laws, which can sometimes impose even stricter restrictions on the agreement. Thus, in contemplating newer models of alignment, appropriate due diligence must always precede adaptation.

However, with the completion of thorough vetting, the compliance and legal challenges, while still present, should be mitigated significantly. With this in mind, there are no legal restrictions on even the newer forms of alignment. However, they must be structured to comply with the regulations in various relevant areas of the working relationship, especially the economic arrangements between the hospital and the physician group. This matter is even more important as we shift to what is, for some, the more nebulous process of sharing risk and then rewarding based on this shared risk.

In summary, be aware that alignment has expanded to include several new structures, affording physicians and hospitals more options that will meet their go-forward needs. Also, these alignment models are adapting to serve as an effective base for clinical integration. Instead of having alignment models that reward production only, most alignment models today (whether they are a PSA or employment or another alternative) include both productivity-based and non-production incentives. These non-production incentives, while sometimes the minority of compensation initially, then have the ability to scale over time, as risk-based contracting increases and the parties shift their focus to value, as opposed to production.

Thus, while many of the "first generation" alignment models (typically defined as those existing between 2005 and 2015) lacked true symmetry in terms of both parties' goals, this disparity is being rectified in the "second generation" models now coming into existence. Second generation models tend to seek a "happy medium" between hospital and physician control, better align economic incentives, more clearly define expectations for behaviors, and add a laser-like focus on value.

Overall, the alignment models continue to adapt to meet market demands and pressures and likely will continue to evolve even further over the next five years.

EDUCATING PHYSICIANS

It is not uncommon for physicians to accuse hospitals of moving slowly, and it is not unusual for hospitals to assert that physician behaviors can be difficult to change. While there is likely some truth to both points, the reality is that transitioning to a value-based environment requires all parties to overcome any historical perspectives they have about the other, and to the extent those biases are warranted, to improve upon them and function more efficiently and effectively.

For organizations to succeed with clinical integration, physicians need to be the front-line leaders who are driving change. In fact, the FTC definition of clinical integration *mandates* physician leadership. So, if an organization wants to pursue clinical integration—the pathway to success in the value-based environment—then physician leadership is an absolute requirement. But how do you get physicians involved even as participants, much less to serve as leaders? If physician engagement is imperative, how does one accomplish it? Managing physician engagement requires the following:

- Establishment of clear goals with the input of physicians (both qualitative and quantitative);
- Real-time data that allows physicians the ability to compare their performance against national and network standards;
- Transparent reporting that allows for continuous process improvements;
- Physicians being willing to participate in contemporary healthcare methods (i.e., evidence-based, best practice care guidelines, population health management, etc.); and
- Analysis of physician referral patterns—both in and out of network—to determine potential for physician reinforcement.

So, what will motivate physicians to be engaged? The primary drivers of physician engagement can be summarized as follows:

- Decision Making Roles
  - It is appropriate to involve physicians in decision making that affects outcomes, their clinical practice methodology, and overall administrative functions.
  - These decisions may include designing compensation incentives, developing quality metrics, creating care processes, driving process improvement, etc.
- Results of Reimbursement
  - As MACRA/MIPS becomes increasingly important to physicians' total reimbursement, it is likely that they will be more willing to participate in activities that drive success under these systems.
  - Thus, organizations should be transparent about reimbursement rates, payment adjustments, and the transition process.
- Voice in Operational Strategy
  - Physicians who link their economic future to an organization's performance want a say in its strategy and execution, and more importantly, are the key driving force behind achieving many economic goals.
  - As such, organizations should be responsive to physician input and make actions/decisions that reflect physicians' priorities.
- Physician Leadership Opportunities
  - A key function of driving engagement is placing physician constituents in leadership positions.
  - Organizations should identify physician champions to lead projects and reward/compensate them for their time.
  - They should foster development of leadership skills and provide opportunities to network with leadership.
- Relationships with Other Providers and Organizations
  - A critical function for integration is sharing resources and creating economies of scale across disparate practices, service lines, providers, etc., (aggregating patients, technology or support needs, specialty services, etc.).
  - This initiative will create a more collaborative continuum of care within the organization.

With an understanding of the drivers for physician engagement, an organization is ready to take action in a way that resounds with physicians and may impact their behavior significantly. Some approaches to improve engagement include the following:

- Develop a shared mission and vision.
  - Develop a philosophy of mutual benefit and shared vision.
  - Strive for transparency from upper management down.

—Solicit meaningful physician input early and often, and then act on it.

—Engage physicians in balancing business and clinical priorities.

—Set realistic goals together and go for early wins.

- Nurture physician leaders.

—Identify, mentor, and educate physician leaders.

—Invest in physician leaders.

—Reward physicians in ways they value.

—Attend a leadership conference together or hire a coach to complete leadership training on-site.

—Get to know physicians on a personal level—conduct one-to-one meetings.

- Communicate effectively.

—Ask questions and ensure that any grievances are addressed quickly.

—Use multiple forms of communication, multiple times.

—Manage physicians by walking around—listen and learn.

—Determine the motivation behind physicians, and work to create incentives that match.

- Capture and share data.

—Implement processes that help determine what data is to be collected and how.

—Use data as the platform for discussions on improving care and lowering costs.

—Foster trusting relationships by sharing data frequently and broadly.

—Encourage physicians to use data to make decisions.

- Develop metrics and hold physicians accountable.

—Ensure that physicians are a part of creating the metrics (quality, cost, patient satisfaction, etc.).

—Make metrics specific to each specialty and/or sub-specialty (depending on the size of the organization).

—Utilize physicians to meet with colleagues who fail to meet these measures.

—Tie specific incentives to these metrics (i.e., compensation, service line improvement initiatives, medical directorships, etc.).

- Work toward clinical integration. (See Figure 3.2 for further information regarding various launching points on the journey to integration.)

—Establish a collaborative method of delivering care, regardless of the format in which you pursue clinical integration.

—Involve as many physicians as possible (employed, community, etc.).

—Determine a method that best meets your needs—not all organizations should immediately pursue an ACO or CIN.

In summary, be aware that the key to participating successfully in any value-based reimbursement model is to ensure there is significant support for these efforts from the physicians of the organization. For example, if an organization

Aligned and Engaged	Aligned and Unengaged	Independent and Engaged	Independent and Unengaged
•This is the best starting point for your organization and should provide you with a relatively easy transition. •Still, there are likely significant infrastructure and operational considerations prior to fully integrating.	•While this is still a good starting point, as likely your providers share similar management, etc., there needs to be significant focus on why engagement remains low. •Before proceeding, the organization should seek to improve their provider engagement, ensuring there isn't a larger systemic issue.	•Alignment is not necessary for clinical integration – in fact, there are various models for clinical integration that incorporate physician-only or hospital-to-community provider organizations. •The engagement will be critical for gaining trust among the independent providers, especially when it comes to sharing data.	•While this is not the ideal position to be in, it does provide significant opportunities for the organization to "start from scratch" and begin building a highly collaborative clinically integrated model. •However, as with the others, this will take significant investments of time and resources to effectuate.

FIGURE 3.2. Using Physician Engagement and Alignment to Drive Integration

pursues a bundled payment, it will take substantial cooperation from each provider within the bundled payment model to make sure they are working collaboratively with all other providers. Further, these providers must then be dedicated to providing care at the highest quality for the lowest cost possible, while taking into consideration the other aspects of care previously or still to be delivered.

Thus, organizations should first view their organization's current engagement before pursuing such a contract. If the commitment is notably low, significant focus should be on increasing physician engagement across the organization. Then, the organizations should introduce these initiatives to their provider leadership and garner feedback, consistently leaning on these leaders for support and guidance. Overall, if the physicians do not agree to participate in these activities, the initiative inevitably will fail.

RVUS WITHIN ALIGNMENT MODELS

As discussed more extensively in Chapter 6, there continues to be a role for RVUs within alignment models today, and for the foreseeable future. The role of RVUs is two-fold: a measure of production, and a factor in compensation.

RVUs historically have been seen as an accurate representation of physician productivity in that they reward the effort expended and are based on a common standard. Physicians have typically appreciated that RVUs provide credit for services performed when collections did not—as in the case of uninsured or under-insured patients for which no revenue was received. Hospitals appreciated having a standard that applied across specialties and that covered the majority of services rendered by providers (thus, sparing them the effort and potential headache of having to create independently a rubric by which all physicians were to be measured).

As discussed in detail in Chapter 4, compensation in today's alignment structures include significantly less focus on productivity and significantly more focus on patient satisfaction, cost of care, efficiency, good citizenship, and other non-production measures. More often, compensation is being impacted by not just process measures but true outcomes measures. However, when production is included in the compensation model, the near-exclusive production measure used is RVUs.

In summary, be aware that while RVUs will continue to have a role within alignment models as a measure of production, as alignment shifts to integration, the prevalence of RVUs as a factor in compensation is likely to decrease.

CONCLUSION

Remember when everyone thought Diagnosis-Related Groups were utterly revolutionary—out of the box and crazy? Well, someday in the future, it is likely that our successors will be laughing at our apprehensions about this "new-fangled" value-based payment system that is now upon us. But, hopefully, they will appreciate the manner in which we responded to it, which is the emphasis we placed on "working together" to ensure our collective success. Physician-hospital alignment offers an effective vehicle to unite parties and focus their efforts on shared goals and is indeed one of the best ways to respond to the value-based environment.

The rise of fee-for-value reimbursement has created an industry-wide call to action, with MACRA having led the way. However, it is essential to be proactive rather than reactive, without *overreacting*. Alignment is an excellent avenue to mitigate numerous economic, strategic, and operational concerns. Thus, private groups and health systems should consider a pluralistic approach to alignment at present and beyond. And, as population health management becomes more of a focal point, alignment will be even more elevated, but integration will become essential. Ultimately, it is balancing and then maximizing physician-hospital alignment, clinical integration, and physician engagement that will yield all parties the greatest possible success in the new wave of reimbursement.

The four "starting points" for transitioning your provider base toward true integration can vary, as noted below. However, the ultimate goal is for an organization to have providers who are *engaged*, whether they are aligned or independent. Engaged providers will yield the greatest chance of success in any integrated structure.

CHAPTER 4

Compensation in a Value-Based Reimbursement World

The use of wRVUs as a form of productivity measurement is a standard practice across the healthcare industry. Compensation methods are shifting from volume-based metrics, such as collections and gross charges, toward a productivity-based distribution. wRVUs are an objective and efficient way to record and report productivity on an individual physician level, and they can be applied universally.

The focus of wRVUs is the services the physician personally performs. Additionally, wRVUs do not factor in poor payer mix or billing/collections inefficiency that may be present in the healthcare setting. The continual use of wRVUs as the primary measure of productivity is one of the purest ways to measure productivity when contemplating physician compensation models.

As the healthcare environment evolves and there continues to be a greater focus on factors other than productivity within physician compensation models, it will become more important to build these incentives into existing compensation arrangements. With the changing reimbursement environment come challenges to the shift in physician compensation from being derived purely from productivity to the inclusion of performance measures. Performance incentives commonly include quality, patient satisfaction and citizenship, cost controls, and coding and compliance, among others, and are more subjective than wRVUs. Therefore, more compensation is "at risk" relative to these components. Unlike wRVUs, productivity incentives are much harder to track and are not equitable in terms of primary and specialty care.

This chapter focuses on the impact of value-based metrics and how wRVU-based compensation models are changing as the focus on value-based reimbursement grows. Specifically, we look at the changing physician compensation models in both private practices and hospital-employed settings.

PRIVATE PRACTICE VS. HOSPITAL EMPLOYMENT

Physician compensation is a core focus in both private practices and hospital employment, but the dynamics of each situation are different. The key difference is the funds available to the physician for compensation.

In private practice, funds that can be paid out to the physicians as compensation are limited because the pool of compensation dollars is derived based on the collections generated by the practice, less their overhead. Thus, if a practice generates $2,000,000 in profits before physician compensation, this is the amount that can be paid out to the physicians. In the next year, if the profit before physician compensation drops to $1,800,000, the physicians, as a group, experience a 10% decline in their compensation.

The focus on physician compensation within a private practice, therefore, is on determining the most equitable manner to allocate the available dollars among the physicians. Of course, the available dollars are influenced by how well revenue is maximized (or not) and expenses are controlled.

Typically, employed physicians are compensated differently than partner physicians, though this is not always the case. Employed physicians often remain employed for only a few years until they become partners. During this period, they often experience some guaranteed compensation while they build their practice, and then they transition to some sort of "base plus" productivity model. Here, they still receive some level of guaranteed compensation with an opportunity to earn additional incentive compensation. The partner physicians share in the profits before physician compensation. The models can take on a variety of forms, some of which we will explain in this chapter.

The situation is quite different in hospital employment in that the physicians' compensation in employment is not confined solely to the profits generated in the practice. Due to a variety of factors that exist in hospital employment, including a less desirable payer mix, higher overhead, and the lack of ability to expand the practice from an ancillary services perspective, most hospital-employed physicians experience some level of loss after their compensation is considered. Thus, compensation is based more on fair market value and what is commercially reasonable than only what the practice can afford to pay in terms of breaking even.

The key question, then, becomes: what variables should the compensation model include that are most appropriate in providing market-based compensation and that can be justified as commercially reasonable?

Private Practice

While operationally similar to hospital-employed physician groups in many respects, the factors influencing physician compensation can differ significantly. While hospital-employed groups are focused much more on "market-based compensation," private practices solely focus on profitability, as their ability to compensate their physicians is limited to what is left over after all expenses are paid. The movement to value-based reimbursement is complicating this situation even further.

To unpack this concept a bit more, in many respects private practice compensation models are the easiest to adapt to the value-based realm. As Figure 4.1 shows, in the private practice profit and loss statement, the addition of value-based reimbursement does not alter the model, as these other forms of reimbursement are treated as revenue.

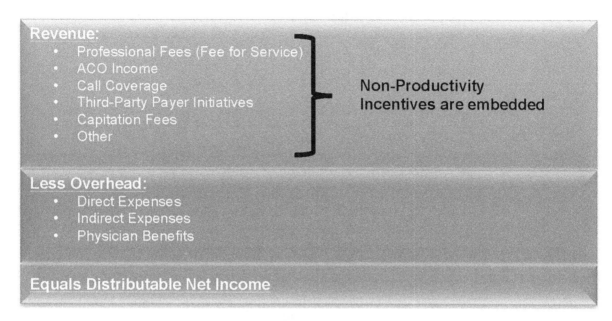

Revenue:
- Professional Fees (Fee for Service)
- ACO Income
- Call Coverage
- Third-Party Payer Initiatives
- Capitation Fees
- Other

} Non-Productivity Incentives are embedded

Less Overhead:
- Direct Expenses
- Indirect Expenses
- Physician Benefits

Equals Distributable Net Income

FIGURE 4.1. Private Practice Profit and Loss Statement

As illustrated, the method used in determining the profit pool in which physician compensation is distributed follows the typical structure of revenue less expenses. New forms of reimbursement can replace professional fee revenue with no change to the overall model. The objective of private practices now is to manage expenses based on the various forms of revenue available for generation.

While this sounds simple, rarely is it this easy. For example, as the revenue streams transition toward value-based arrangements, this affects every facet of practice operations. First, the practice must ensure that the total revenue pool is not decreasing. Specifically, if fee-for-service revenue is diminishing, both in terms of the amount per encounter, but also as a percentage of the practice's overall revenue, the practice must focus on finding new sources of revenue. These sources could take on many forms, such as value-based arrangements with payers, affiliations/arrangements with local health systems, etc. The key is that if revenue decreases, so too will the compensation pool, given the largely fixed nature of practice overhead.

Then, the practice must focus on its overhead. For instance, as the revenue sources change, so too will the expense structures. As an example, a primary care practice may need to invest in certain population health tools and/or add care coordinators/navigators to help staff function properly under capitated or semi-capitated arrangements. Thus, it is important for the overhead structure of the practice to also change as the revenue sources change.

Finally, and most pertinent to this text, is the compensation methodology. Historically, private practices have frequently taken an "eat-what-you-kill" mentality, which is that the individual provider productivity has driven the compensation equation to a large extent. A common compensation model would be 100% of professional fee collections flowing to each physician and then expenses being allocated as partially fixed and partially variable based on the individual decisions of that practice. So, productivity is significant in that the more revenue generated, the more drops to the bottom line, assuming all practice costs are covered.

The challenge that a shift in focus brings is that productivity may not be the only driver of revenue going forward. A great example is reimbursement under the Merit-based Incentive Payment System (MIPS) in a private practice setting. Historically, a physician saw a Medicare patient, provided a service, and got paid at the Medicare reimbursement rate for that service. Now, the same equation would apply, but the rate at which the physician received payment would vary based on how well the physician performed with respect to the MIPS metrics. So, a physician might decide that doing more is a means to an end. And, if he is not performing well relative to MIPS scores, it may be more advantageous financially for him to find ways to improve the care he is providing to a lower volume of patients. In other words, ultimately, doing a better job for fewer patients could lead to more reimbursement than would performing at a lower level of quality for more patients.

Another example of the MIPS model is a physician who is involved in a shared savings arrangement. She may realize more value by dedicating some time to the programmatic efforts in the shared savings arrangement versus seeing one additional patient that day. This means that the achievement of shared savings at the end of the year may be worth more than increased volume.

So, instead of a situation where the focus of a physician's time was evident—increasing volume—this element is no longer the case. There may indeed be revenue-generating activities that are driven by factors other than increased volume, which are essential activities to identify within a practice's income distribution plan. Thus, a private practice may need to tweak its model to ensure that all physicians are focused on revenue-generating activities, which may include more than simply increasing fee-for-service volume. Practices can go about this in different ways. Following are some examples of ways in which private practices have incorporated value-based incentives into their compensation plan.

Maintain the Status Quo

Some practices have taken the stance that they will not change anything, despite the changing healthcare landscape. Depending on how significant the change is in their specific market, this plan may or may not work. Thus, if there is a significant push toward value-based reimbursement in their market, the failure to adapt will likely hurt the practice economically because there will be a misalignment between what is driving reimbursement and the incentives of the physicians.

In other markets where there is minimal change, the practice may do fine with not changing the compensation paradigm. This outcome may be because the changes are immaterial or the pain and disruption in redeveloping the income distribution plan outweigh the economic impact of lost value-based incentives, if any. This issue is comparable to physician practices that made similar decisions about electronic health records.

Another way such a plan could work is if the value-based incentives are all tracked/measured on an individual physician basis. If such is the case, the "eat-what-you-kill" compensation arrangement would still work, as the individual physicians would be incentivized to maximize the various sources of their revenue.

Carve-Out as Ancillary

Another approach that private practices take with respect to value-based services is to carve them out of the normal practice activities and treat them more like an ancillary service. To set the stage, let's say a practice has a physical therapy (PT) service line. PT is a core part of their business but functions separately from the rest of the practice—separate revenue streams, expense structures, etc. In such a case, the owners of the practice may share equally in the profits they generate. Certain value-based activities, such as the creation of an accountable care organization (ACO) or participation in a bundled payment program, could be treated similarly. This method likely only makes sense when the physicians are indirectly involved in the activities, and there are very discreet revenue streams and overhead items associated with the value-based activity.

Direct Incorporation into Compensation Model

Some practices incorporate value-based incentives directly into their compensation model. This means that a portion of the overall funds available for distribution is not tied to fee-for-service revenue generation but value-based activities, which can take many different forms. One example is a practice that distributes most of its available dollars using targeted percentages of collections. In such a case, physicians producing below the 40th percentile of wRVUs are paid at 45% of collections; those between the 40th and 60th percentile are paid at 50% of collections; and physicians producing above the 60th percentile are paid at 55% of collections.

The expectation is that this approach will only distribute 90% to 95% of available compensation. The rest of the compensation goes into a performance pool that is divided equally based on the number of physicians in the medical group. This defines the performance incentive opportunity. The amount that is then paid out is based on each respective physician's performance against an established scorecard. Any remaining funds are rolled over into the following year's distribution pool.

Another example is a practice that allocates all or a portion of its group overhead (similar to MSO-type costs) based on performance against an established scorecard. Physicians who perform very well receive a lower allocation of overhead, whereas physicians who perform poorly experience a higher allocation of overhead. The rationale for this methodology is that the group overhead touches all physicians and, therefore, is a central point in the income distribution plan to tie group-based incentives.

Other groups continue to use an "eat-what-you-kill" approach but withhold a portion of earned compensation (for example, 10%) and pay it out based only on the achievement of certain pre-established value-based metrics. The challenge with this approach is that the physicians perceive themselves as having to earn the compensation twice: once by actually performing the work and then by meeting the established performance metrics. While this plan seems onerous, many elements of a similar strategy exist within the MIPS model.

wRVUs in Private Practice Models

While the model structures are changing, as referenced above, wRVUs are still frequently utilized in private practice models. As noted, wRVUs are considered as the most objective metric and, thus, are the predominant allocation tool in determining individual physician compensation in the private practice realm. wRVUs are not used as the primary driver of compensation in private practices as they do not always translate directly to dollars.

In private practice where "cash is king," the focus is primarily on cash collections in terms of driving compensation. However, as noted, wRVUs can still be used to allocate cash collections, overhead, etc., among the individual physicians. Private practices also commonly blend wRVUs with other productivity metrics, such as collections and/or gross charges. The blending of productivity metrics is appropriate when services result in high collections but have a disproportionate wRVU value or vice versa. In this instance, using only wRVUs as a performance metric could be a deterrent from performing these low wRVU value services. Alternatively, using only collections may push providers to want only to work in the offices where the payer mix is best. Under a blending scenario, the metrics used are weighted either equally or with one metric weighted more heavily. It is up to the practice to study the effects of potential distribution plans to determine how best to weight metrics and allocate funds.

In summary, with respect to private practices, the compensation models are changing, primarily driven by the new forms of reimbursement that are tied more to value than pure volume. The use of wRVUs in private practice compensation models has not been impacted by this change, with their role in private practice models largely being a means of allocating compensation available within the group, as opposed to being the sole source of driving compensation for each physician.

HOSPITAL-EMPLOYED SETTINGS

Over the last decade, the physician market has changed dramatically, with many physicians joining health systems as employees. This shift has had a dramatic effect on compensation strategies. What has been most notable about the change in compensation strategies as physicians have moved into hospital employment is that the focus is no longer solely on practice financial performance but relies on other measures of productivity. An interesting point about this shift is that a private practice model tends to work very well in a changing reimbursement environment.

This matter can be considered in relation to the discussion on private practice models and their adaptation to value-based reimbursement, above. Prior to value-based reimbursement, the calculation was a rather simple one. Professional fee revenue less direct expenses equaled physician compensation. With new forms of revenue, the calculation becomes a bit more complicated, but it still follows the same pattern. That is, revenue less expenses equals physician compensation. What is nice about this approach is that the model structure accepts all forms of reimbursement. ACO distributions can replace professional fee revenue easily with no change in the model structure. The key is in managing expenses based on the various forms of revenue available for generation. Thus, the model is very adaptable to moving toward value-based reimbursement.

The central challenge with a private practice-style model is that it is the hardest to implement in a hospital-employed environment for a variety of factors, one of which is the higher expense structure in hospital-employed settings due to an escalation in wage scales, occupancy costs, and other overhead items. Further, the payer mix can change, which results in less professional fee revenue. These and other factors can end in the private practice-style model not resulting in market compensation and thereby being perceived as untenable in a hospital-employed environment. Rarely do we see such a model implemented in a hospital-employed setting.

As a result, there is no simple formula to pull value-based metrics into a hospital-employed compensation arrangement. Even the simplest structures can present significant challenges. As an example, a hospital implemented an $8,000 performance incentive opportunity per physician. For a physician making $200,000, this represented 4% of their compensation. For a physician making $400,000, this represented 2% of their total compensation. Thus, in the grand scheme of the overall compensation arrangement, the value associated with this provision was small, but the hospital's compensation committee spent more time dealing with the dynamics of this component than anything else.

The discussions were about what metrics should be tracked, where the data are available and accurate for those metrics, how often the data should/could be reported, how much value should be tied to the metrics, whether the metrics are meaningful, to which specialties they should apply, etc. When the dynamics of this model are juxtaposed to a simple wRVU-based compensation formula that has limited moving parts/pieces, the challenge of implementing is onerous.

Impact on wRVU Models

There is an overwhelming sense in the market that as value-based reimbursement ramps up, wRVU-based models will go by the wayside. For the foreseeable future, wRVUs will have a place for many years to come in hospital-employed compensation models. This matter is especially the case for specialty care, where other than certain episodic initiatives, such as the Comprehensive Care for Joint Replacement or certain bundled payment pilots, fee-for-service reimbursement still predominates. Even other programs that apply to specialty care physicians, such as MIPS (discussed above and in earlier chapters), are still heavily productivity-based (read wRVU-based).

If wRVUs remain the primary means of reimbursement to align incentives, the compensation structure should be no different. Thus, until the market moves to a largely fully capitated model wherein the capitation payments also include specialty care services, wRVU-based production likely will continue to play a role in the compensation strategy. Though this is occurring in certain markets, such as Vermont, it is not the norm throughout the industry/country.

While primary care is somewhat different, wRVUs still play a role. For primary care, wRVUs are being balanced out by a focus on patient panels. Patient panels typically are defined as unique patients seen by a physician in the past 18 months. A standard panel for a primary care physician averages around 1,800 unique patients. Panel-based models are synonymous with capitation, wherein the revenue generated is not necessarily based on how much you do but on how many patients you manage. While there are pockets of capitation throughout the market, it is not yet a dominant reimbursement mechanism. Thus, fully moving a primary care model to panel size would be a bit premature. The use of panel incentives in compensation arrangements is addressed in later chapters.

Once again, the incentive structure reverts to wRVUs, as this is still driving reimbursement. Even if we find ourselves in a fully capitated market, that dynamic does not mean that wRVUs will go away. While wRVUs may not be the primary driver of incentive in a compensation model, it would still be reasonable to use them to measure what a physician is doing for the population of patients he or she is managing. Thus, wRVUs, while their use is evolving, will continue to play a role for the foreseeable future.

The MIPS that is a part of the Medicare Access and CHIP Reauthorization Act (MACRA) will undoubtedly impact wRVU-based compensation strategies in the future. Figure 4.2 illustrates the typical wRVU-based structure in its most simplistic form pre-MIPS. The model could be tiered, etc., but, at its root, it consisted of wRVUs being multiplied by a conversion factor/rate per wRVU.

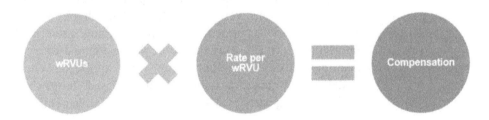

FIGURE 4.2. wRVU-Based Structure

The formula was rather simple. wRVUs were multiplied by a market-based compensation per wRVU ratio to derive compensation. Thus, the only factor influencing compensation was how much a physician did, measured in wRVUs. With MIPS, this is no longer the case. While MIPS still focuses on how much a physician does, reimbursement is ultimately impacted by how well he performs the work. Thus, there are additional hurdles to jump through that affect ultimate reimbursement. In the context of a wRVU-based compensation model, the impact of MIPS can be illustrated in Figure 4.3.

The equation is similar, but instead of the rate per wRVU being a constant, it is influenced by how well a physician performs in certain key non-productive areas. Thus, MIPS is a game changer with respect to reimbursement and should have the same effect on compensation arrangements.

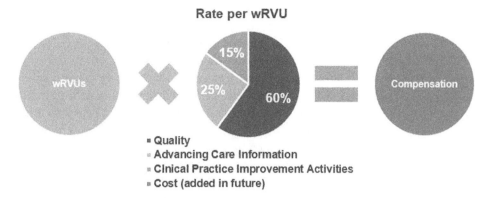

FIGURE 4.3. Rate per wRVU

The effects of MIPS and other value-based arrangements are causing health systems to redesign their compensation arrangements in a variety of ways that focus mostly on rebalancing the emphasis on production and performance. The appropriate balance is largely predicated on local reimbursement dynamics, with more aggressive markets pushing health systems to put more in the value/performance bucket, with the opposite not moving as quickly in this direction.

Overall, the balance of production and performance in the primary care realm tends to be a 70/30 to 85/15 split, with the former being the production focus and the latter being the performance/value focus. With specialty care, the split is more in the range of 85/15 to 95/5, with less of a focus on the value-based piece. This calculation is driven primarily by the market and less activity in the performance/value space for these specialties.

Incorporation of Value-Based Components

The incorporation of value-based components is impacted by the specialty involved, with the key consideration being whether the physicians are hospital-based or ambulatory/surgical physicians. In the following section, we articulate how models are taking shape in the value-based world in these two large subsets of the physician population.

Hospital-Based Physicians

A prime differentiating factor for hospital-based physicians is that their compensation is based primarily on time worked versus productivity (wRVUs, collections, etc.) generated. Thus, the shift to value-based reimbursement is not as dynamic for them, but given the critical role they play in driving the performance of the hospital, it is essential to integrate value-based elements into their compensation structure.

Often, this initiative involves reducing their time-based compensation slightly wherein value-based incentives can be incorporated. Given the time-based nature of their compensation arrangements, there is not an infinite amount of tolerance for reducing the base level of compensation, but performance incentives should not be entirely an add-on. Meaning, the target should be achieving market-based compensation and ensuring there is an appropriate balance between what is guaranteed based on time worked and what is tied to incentives.

Frequently, we see a target of 5% to 15% of compensation being tied to incentives. Thus, as a simple example, a hospitalist may be paid $1,450 per 12-hour shift as base compensation, with the opportunity to earn an additional $150 per shift, depending on the achievement of certain performance metrics. Thus, the target for market-based compensation is the total compensation opportunity of $1,600. The same approach can apply on an hourly basis.

Alternatively, the hospital may simply decide to apportion a total amount of compensation per year to performance incentives. For example, a full-time physician may have the opportunity to earn $25,000 per year in performance incentives. If such is the approach, it is important to ensure that the baseline compensation for time worked and the performance incentives equate to market-based compensation when considered in their totality.

So, the adaptation of hospital-based compensation models for value-based incentives is rather straight-forward with the primary focus being on what metrics to incentivize. Structurally, the transition is relatively simple.

Ambulatory/Surgical Physicians

There are infinite possibilities in adapting compensation arrangements for the value-based world in the ambulatory/surgical realm. Below, instead of highlighting overarching model options, we focus on the main concepts that should be of consideration in any model structure.

STRUCTURE OF WRVU-BASED MODEL

Within the market, there are many wRVU models and levels of complexity. These can range from single-tier approaches wherein all wRVUs are simply paid at the same rate, to multi-tiered approaches. The key focus should be keeping the structure as simple as possible but still driving the objectives desired by the organization.

One option that is moderately complex is a three-tier model. In this model, Tier One is a sort of "penalty" tier, paying at a lower rate per wRVU. The intention here is to recognize the cost of lower-producing physicians. Figure 4.4 illustrates how we typically would structure the model currently in place.

FIGURE 4.4. Three-tier Model Illustration			
Tier	Low	High	Rate
One (if production is below 4,500)	--	4,500	$36.00
Two (If production is above 4,500)	--	5,500	$40.00
Three	5,500	--	$45.00

In this approach, the Tier Two rate is the "targeted rate" (further discussion to follow), with the Tier One rate being 10% below the Tier Two rate, and the Tier Three rate being 10% above the Tier Two rate. Tier Three applies only incrementally. Thus, in this approach, lower-producing physicians are paid less per wRVU. The key in the model is setting the breakpoint between Tier One and Tier Two at the "minimum work standard" of the practice—the level that is desired of all physicians. The breakpoint between Tier One and Tier Two can be set around the median. Further, the Tier Three breakpoint can be set at the 65th or 75th percentile.

Such a structure as is outlined above is just one approach of many, but recognizes the cost of lower-producing physicians, as well as rewards higher-producing physicians.

ESTABLISHING THE RATE PER WRVU

A key consideration within the productivity incentive structure is defining the rate per wRVU. Once a revised model structure is established, a next key step is defining the economics for that model.

Rates per wRVU are set considering a variety of factors, but they often hover near the median. The rationale is that a rate per wRVU near the median results in the best alignment between pay and productivity. Rates per wRVU outside of this range are not representative of normal practice situations. For example, a rate per wRVU at the 75th percentile is likely a new physician who just started but is still ramping up, or a physician in a rural market wherein there will never be enough productivity to keep her busy. Figure 4.5 illustrates this concept.

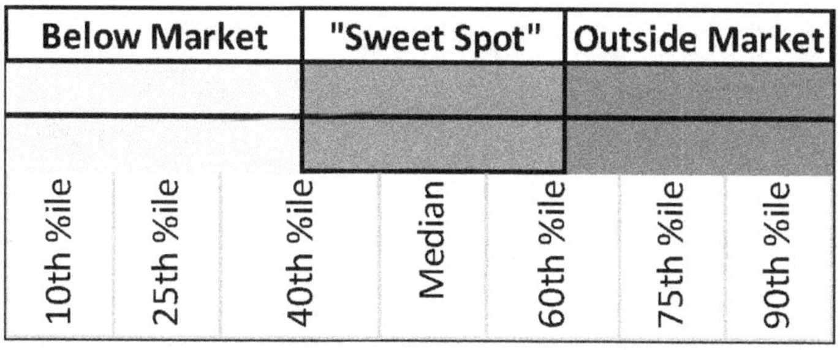

Below Market			"Sweet Spot"		Outside Market	
10th %ile	25th %ile	40th %ile	Median	60th %ile	75th %ile	90th %ile

FIGURE 4.5. Market Rates/Ranges

Using the median rate per wRVU tends to align compensation and productivity and is not necessarily a representation of the level of compensation as illustrated in the Figure 4.6.

Rate per wRVU < Median = wRVU > Compensation

Rate per wRVU > Median = wRVU < Compensation

Rate per wRVU = Median = wRVU = Compensation

FIGURE 4.6. National Market Data Relationships					
wRVUs	Mkt %ile	TCC/ wRVU	Mkt %ile	Total Cash Compensation	Mkt %ile
3,822	25th %ile	$48.45	40th %ile	$185,168	20th %ile
4,754	Median	$48.45	40th %ile	$230,322	45th %ile
5,761	75th %ile	$48.45	40th %ile	$279,109	66th %ile
3,822	25th %ile	$51.19	Median	$195,648	25th %ile
4,754	Median	$51.19	Median	$243,357	52nd %ile
5,761	75th %ile	$51.19	Median	$294,906	72nd %ile
3,822	25th %ile	$56.64	60th %ile	$216,495	36th %ile
4,754	Median	$56.64	60th %ile	$269,287	62nd %ile
5,761	75th %ile	$56.64	60th %ile	$326,328	79th %ile

As illustrated in Figure 4.7, all incentives should be carved out of the target rate per wRVU rather than added on top of the target rate per wRVU. This best practice ensures that the model structure is being driven by a value that will produce total compensation aligned with productivity. Further, it is consistent with market data wherein the benchmarks represent all forms of cash compensation, not just wRVU productivity. The meaning here is that the market data represent quality incentives, call pay, etc., in addition to wRVU-based pay.

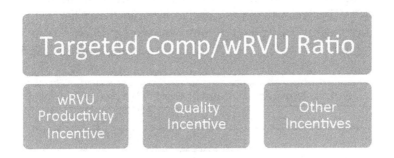

FIGURE 4.7. Incentive Carve-out Targets

While best practice is having some level of consistency in establishing the targeted compensation per wRVU ratio across specialties, the allocation of value does not necessarily have to be the same for all specialties. Thus, it may make sense to put more value in the quality/performance incentive for primary care versus specialty care. As an illustration, consider the chart in Figure 4.8.

In Figure 4.8, for primary care, 80% of pay is in the wRVU-based bucket, with more in this bucket for specialty care. The other key consideration is that the movement to have more value in buckets other than wRVU productivity can be gradual over time. Consider the illustration in Figure 4.9 concerning the current approach versus a three-year transition strategy.

While the goal may be to get more into the quality bucket, it may not be feasible on day one due to system limitations and the newness of quality incentives.

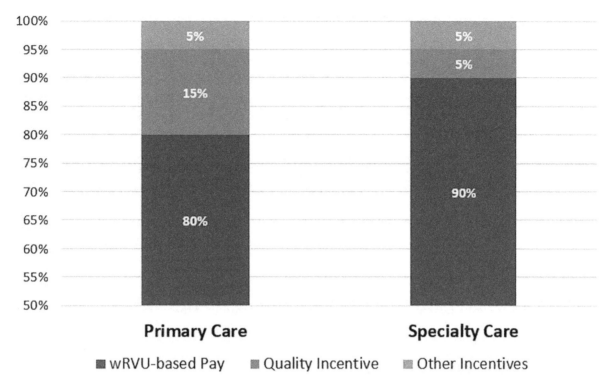

FIGURE 4.8. Incentives for Primary Care vs Specialty Care

FIGURE 4.9. wRVU-based Buckets Three-year Transition Strategy				
	Current	Year One	Year Two	Year Three
Production	95.00%	90.00%	85.00%	80.00%
Quality	0.00%	5.00%	10.00%	15.00%
Other	5.00%	5.00%	5.00%	5.00%
Clinical TCC	**100.00%**	**100.00%**	**100.00%**	**100.00%**

However, it could be more feasible as 1) the reimbursement environment continues to change, and 2) comfort with this type of incentive structure increases.

PERFORMANCE (NON-PRODUCTIVITY) INCENTIVES

As the healthcare environment evolves, there continues to be a greater focus on factors other than productivity within compensation models. A key desire of many hospitals is to build these incentives into the existing compensation arrangement, with many hospitals still having little to no value incorporated into these realms. The non-productivity incentive can be structured in a variety of ways. The key points of focus relative to performance incentives are: structure, value, and metrics. Below, we outline several options for further consideration.

Structural Options

Generally, the best practice is using the allocation of value concept to establish the economics of the performance incentive. By this, we mean taking the targeted rate per wRVU times the value allocated to the performance incentive and then multiplying this by wRVUs generated. As an example, if the targeted rate is $50.00, and 10% is allocated to this component, and the physician generated 4,000 wRVUs, the performance incentive opportunity would be $20,000. Once the economics are in place, there are many structure options, as noted below.

Fixed Dollar Amount: One approach is to target a fixed dollar amount per physician—for example, $15,000 per physician to fund non-productivity incentives. The physician may earn part or all of the incentive based on the scoring of the non-productivity metrics. If pursued, the total performance incentive opportunity would be calculated for the entire practice using the allocation of value concept, and this would guide the per-FTE fixed dollar amount that is ultimately established.

Allocation Based on Panel Size: Another approach to primary care is to calculate the total performance incentive opportunity at the primary care level and then allocate this amount based on each physician's panel size. The rationale here is that panel size is an indication of the patients a physician manages, and therefore, it would make sense to reward that physician based on quality, using the panel as the basis. Here, a physician who has a larger panel size has more opportunity to influence quality than one with a small panel size.

Variable Rate per wRVU: In this approach, we simply let the allocation of value concept play out, with the individual wRVUs dictating the performance incentive opportunity. Thus, higher producers have a larger performance incentive opportunity than lower producers.

The above approaches determine the opportunity associated with this incentive. The actual amount paid should be driven by the physicians' performance with respect to the established incentives. This concept is addressed below.

Value

In our experience, 5%–15% of compensation is often tied to these types of incentives. In most instances, the norm is 10%–15% for primary care and 5%–10% for specialty care. As highlighted earlier, when organizations are new at quality incentives, it is best to start small and build up to higher values, which is typically more accepted by physicians.

Further, if the hospital receives any external quality incentives, such as pay for performance, we recommend that these not be passed directly through to physicians but viewed as a source of revenue to fund the compensation model. This concept is discussed further below.

Metrics

The metrics that are of focus in these incentive structures vary by organization; however, Figure 4.10 outlines some common focus areas (the most common are in bold). It will be important to incorporate the ongoing establishment and management of these metrics into the practice's governance processes. This typically occurs through the creation of a quality committee, which establishes metrics for each specialty and recommends them to the overall compensation committee for approval.

FIGURE 4.10. Table of Metrics	
• **Quality Measures**	• Chart Completion
• **Patient Satisfaction**	• Administrative Adherence
• Expense Control (Practice)	• **Good Citizenship**
• Targeted Cost Savings (Hospital)	• Adoption of EHR
• Coding and Compliance	• Referral Patterns
• Call Coverage	• Medical Home Success

In terms of incorporating the metrics into the compensation arrangement, we recommend the development of a scorecard that has a potential score of 100. The score is then broken down to between two and three quality metrics: patient satisfaction and one or two citizenship metrics. An objective scoring process is then defined for each respective metric. (Note: The three metrics noted in bold—quality measures, patient satisfaction, and good citizenship—are the ones most often used in or applied to the compensation arrangement.)

Ultimately, it is important to ensure that the metrics chosen are meaningful and accurately trackable. Further, there needs to be a balance between the metrics selected and the value assigned. For example, $50,000 in value should not be tied to a single metric nor should $5,000 be tied to 20 metrics, as is addressed below.

Finally, we recommend these incentives be paid out no more often than semi-annually.

TREATMENT OF EXTERNAL INCENTIVES

An added phenomenon with new value-based compensation models is the fact that revenue sources have expanded to include more than just fee-for-service revenue. Now, there are other revenue streams from participation in ACO/CIN activities, shared savings models, government and commercial pay for performance programs, and others. A vital question about these new streams of revenue is what to do with them. In many cases, these programs start out small and then grow. In one year, there may be $500 to $1,000 attributed to a physician for his or her activity in a respective program.

In these instances, health systems have decided to treat these revenue streams as additional compensation and pass them through to the particular physician. While this is not always a problem, in the current environment, two factors have made this approach problematic.

The first challenge is that many compensation models were not designed to accommodate these additional incentives, which gets back to the "top-down" vs. "bottom-up" approach to compensation design discussed earlier. If the compensation model was not designed to have these funds passed through from a fair market value perspective, it could create potential compliance concerns. Remember, the market surveys used for compensation design and benchmarking, i.e., Medical Group Management Association, American Medical Group Association, and Sullivan, Cotter, and Associates, define compensation benchmarks as total cash compensation (TCC)—that is, all forms of compensation that show up on a physician's IRS Form W-2 or K-1. Thus, if a physician is paid quality incentives, they would already be included in the metrics used to define TCC, meaning if the current compensation model is providing market-based compensation, these additional incentives should not necessarily be paid on top of the market-based compensation package.

The second challenge is the differentiation between revenue and compensation. As noted, in many instances, these new forms of revenue are viewed as pass-throughs of additional compensation. There is a big difference here. If value-based reimbursement is replacing fee-for-service reimbursement, then it is problematic to view these types of external incentives as compensation and not revenue. It sets the precedent that 100% of new forms of revenue will be passed through as additional compensation.

Stepping back and considering this statement highlights the problematic nature of the situation. These funds should be viewed as new forms of revenue that then fund both overhead and the current compensation structure. They should not be passed through as additional compensation on top of the existing compensation model. It is incumbent on the health system from a compensation design standpoint to ensure that the incentives in the compensation model are aligned with the incentives that drive value-based reimbursement—similar to what all health systems do with fee-for-service reimbursement in the sense that they use wRVUs or some other form of productivity measure as the primary incentive driver.

Typically, these incentive programs begin with $500–$1,000 per physician, but they can quickly grow to something much more substantial. Further, payers often pay these funds as a true incentive at the onset of a program, then quickly reduce fee-for-service reimbursement wherein to stay whole from a historical perspective, these value-based incentives must be captured. The Centers for Medicare and Medicaid Services (CMS) is notorious for structures like this. This phenomenon exacerbates the issues outlined above.

Further, if a health system sets the precedent that these incentives are going to be passed through in the beginning and physicians get comfortable with the notion, changing course later on becomes even more challenging. Thus, it is important to treat these types of incentives correctly from the outset.

BALANCE OF INCENTIVES AND METRICS

Value-based compensation models, by nature, are designed mainly with the premise of focusing on incentives outside of pure production. Thus, much focus is on quality, patient satisfaction, citizenship, cost control, etc. One reason health systems gravitate to production-based models is that they are easy to administer; the data points come from a single system and can be pulled together quite quickly. When metrics outside of production come into the equation, substantial work is required to gather the data for all of the other focus areas and turn them into something meaningful.

This historically was not a significant issue largely because (1) the incentive component was small ($5,000–$15,000), and (2) the focus of the incentive was on less meaningful metrics. This issue is changing in new models wherein (1) the value of the incentive is growing exponentially larger, and (2) the desire is to focus on more meaningful metrics.

As was mentioned earlier, for primary care, it is not uncommon to see health systems want to tie up to 25% of compensation to value-based metrics. With median primary care compensation being around $230,000, this means close to $60,000 can be tied to these metrics. The key is to determine to what these funds should be tied to justify the assigned value. This issue is a significant struggle, as physicians see these incentives as being riskier than production incentives and, therefore, want them tied to something meaningful, but something they can understand, they can track with accurate data, and they can influence directly. They feel that production incentives are largely in their control, meaning they either have the tools necessary to achieve the productivity incentives or they do not.

This is not the case with value-based incentives, and it mostly stems from a lack of data. While health systems spent millions of dollars implementing new medical records programs, this alone has not resulted in a wealth of data that can be used for value-based incentive metrics. The data may be in the programs, but the know-how to extract the data in a meaningful manner may not exist. Thus, health systems often are left with less-than-desirable metrics that they can track accurately or insufficient meaningful metrics that they want to track.

With this in mind, it is important for health systems to "grow into" these incentives. Moving from $5,000 of value tied to value-based metrics to $60,000 tied to value-based metrics overnight may be a lofty goal if the infrastructure is not there to support the move. While the $60,000 or more may be the ultimate aim, it is important to pace the implementation of these incentives based on the data available; otherwise, buy-in will be difficult.

Further, it is important that health systems not limit themselves only to the incentive they can track or currently are tracking. Rather, they should define what they want to incentivize and determine what is needed to obtain those data. This matter will be more challenging and perhaps delay implementation of these incentives but should pay off in the end as the metrics will drive more change.

Finally, when considering value-based incentives, particularly as the amounts increase, it is important to balance the value of the incentives with the number of incentive metrics. Using an extreme example, it is not reasonable to tie $60,000 of value to a single patient satisfaction metric. At the same time, it is not reasonable to tie $8,000 to 15 different weight metrics. We recommend developing a scorecard that focuses on three or four key quality and patient satisfaction metrics for each specialty, one or two citizenship/access-related metrics, and then another one or two metrics important to group performance. The scorecard should be developed collaboratively by the physicians and the health system and revisited annually to ensure that the metrics are still value-added to the health system.

CONCLUSION

The shift toward value-based reimbursement is having an impact on the physician compensation landscape and as such is affecting both private practices and hospital-employed physicians, albeit in different ways. Part of the challenge that exists today and will exist for years to come is that the reimbursement structure has its feet in both realms: volume and value. The dual realm of volume and value presents challenges in balancing the two from an incentives standpoint. With the uncertainty about which direction the industry will go with reimbursement and what novel types of reimbursement structures will take hold, compensation plans must be nimble and able to shift with the reimbursement structure. Though flexibility is easier said than done, it is a necessity to ensure a successful compensation model that is driving the physicians' behaviors in lockstep with the drivers of reimbursement.

CHAPTER 5

Legal Considerations of the Value-Based Reimbursement Era

This section provides an overview of the legal aspects of RVU-based physician compensation. As is described in other parts of this book, physician compensation may be determined based on several factors, including gross revenue, net collections, RVUs, tiered RVUs, bonuses, and other systems of allocation. Most physician compensation systems involve both a fixed base salary and an additional bonus component.

THE LEGAL BASIS FOR RVUS

Federal law includes numerous references to RVUs. CMS has codified RVUs in the Code of Federal Regulations (CFR) at 42 CFR 414.22. These sections of the CFR describe in detail how to calculate RVUs. CMS also updates RVUs annually as part of the Medicare physician fee schedule rulemaking process. In addition, RVU-based compensation is explicitly recognized in the Stark Law, where productivity bonuses based on RVUs are approved as an appropriate and lawful method to compensate physicians. (See 42 CFR 411.352(i)(3)(i) "Special Rule for productivity bonuses and profit shares.") This rule allows the payment of productivity bonuses based on services performed personally by the physician or based on services incident to those personally performed services.

In addition to the federal laws mentioned above, a number of other legal considerations impact RVU compensation systems: federal anti-kickback laws, federal Advisory Opinions from the Office of the Inspector General, federal tax law, state anti-kickback statutes, state corporate practice of medicine statutes, the Federal False Claims Act, and the Medicare prohibition against assignment of receivables, among others. Each of these areas of law can have an impact on RVU-based physician compensation arrangements. Please note that the Medicaid system provides no guidance in this regard and appears to rely on Medicare.

THE STARK LAW

Of the numerous laws that impact physician compensation, the Stark Law is the most restrictive and the most punitive. The good news is that if a compensation arrangement meets the requirements of the Stark Law or one of its exceptions, then in many cases the requirements of the other laws mentioned above will also be met.

The Stark Law prohibits a physician from making a referral of a designated health service (DHS) to an entity if the physician has a direct or indirect financial relationship with that entity, unless a specific exception applies. Each of the exceptions is specifically worded and requires strict compliance. Further, even practitioners who do not provide a significant volume of Medicare services must comply with the Stark Law if they participate in Medicare at all.

Stark Law does not technically cover those elements of the physician's practice that are outside of Medicare or are not involved in DHSs. However, it is rare for an organization to maintain two separate billing systems and two separate recordkeeping systems, with one for complying with Stark and one for a different compensation system that is not Stark compliant. The Office of Inspector General has indicated that they take a dim view of efforts to game the system and have compensation systems that treat Medicare one way and treat commercially insured payments another way. The result is that virtually every physician compensation arrangement comes within the coverage of the Stark Law for practical reasons or for legal reasons.

The consequences for a financial arrangement that does not achieve strict compliance with a Stark Law exception can be harsh. As a baseline requirement, the involved parties must repay Medicare for any claims for DHS referrals made while the noncompliant arrangement was in place. Further, prohibited referrals made during the noncompliant arrangement may result in substantial fines and penalties. While Stark violations typically do not involve a jail sentence, the civil penalties can be large. For example, CMS may impose a fine of up to $15,000 per claim, regardless of the amount of the claim (be it $1 or $10,000). When those $15,000 fines are multiplied by the thousands of claims for DHS that may be submitted based on referrals by a physician during a tainted arrangement, the fines can become astronomical. These fines have amounted to tens—or even hundreds—of millions of dollars in cases where the reimbursements obtained are comparatively small.

Finally, in serious cases, providers may be excluded from the Medicare program. This is a severe consequence given that few medical practitioners, hospitals, or facilities can survive without participation in the Medicare program. Additionally, exclusion from Medicare normally results in reporting to the National Practitioner Data Bank, loss of malpractice insurance, and little chance of obtaining hospital privileges in the future.

EXCEPTIONS TO THE STARK LAW

While physician compensation arrangements generally qualify as financial relationships governed by the Stark Law, there are two principal exceptions: (1) the bona fide employment exception for W-2 employees; and (2) the personal services arrangement exception for independent contractors. And again, productivity bonuses utilizing RVUs are an explicitly recognized exception under Stark.

To understand how the exceptions work, it is necessary to start with certain definitions under the Stark Law:

1. *Physician.* The definition of physician includes a variety of practitioners, including doctors of medicine, osteopathy, dentists, podiatrists, optometrists, and chiropractors.

2. *Designated Health Services.* The statute includes a list of services that are considered DHS. CMS annually updates and publishes in the Federal Register a specific DHS list that uses CPT codes to more precisely define these terms. The DHS list is as follows:

   a. Clinical laboratory services;

   b. Physical therapy services;

   c. Occupational therapy services;

   d. Radiology services including MRI, CT, and ultrasound;

   e. Radiation therapy services and supplies;

   f. Durable medical equipment and supplies;

   g. Parenteral and enteral nutrients, equipment, and supplies;

   h. Prosthetics, orthotics, prosthetic devices, and supplies;

   i. Home health services;

   j. Outpatient prescription drugs; and

   k. Inpatient and outpatient hospital services.

   Notably, professional services provided in a physician's office are <u>not</u> on the list, nor are surgeries.

3. *Financial Relationship.* A financial relationship under Stark can be a direct or indirect ownership or investment interest, or a direct or indirect compensation arrangement, between a physician and an entity that furnishes DHS. This covers any kind of investment interest, salaries, bonuses, income guarantees, medical director payments and on-call fees, and incentive compensation in any form including RVUs. Further, financial relationships are construed fairly broadly, to include such relationships between DHS entities and physicians' immediate family members such as husbands and wives, parents, children and siblings, and even more distant relations like stepparents, stepchildren, stepsiblings, in-laws, grandparents, and grandchildren and their spouses.

All compensation to physicians pursuant to hospital employment is covered by Stark because employment establishes a financial relationship, and physicians typically refer to their employer hospital. In contrast, to the extent that physician compensation in a medical group does not involve anything that is on the DHS list, that compensation is free of the restrictions that are in the Stark Law. However, the referral of a DHS item by a physician in a medical group is covered by Stark and that list is extensive. As a result of the pervasive coverage of the DHS list, most medical groups structure their compensation arrangements in strict compliance with Stark.

Stark Exception for Bona Fide Employment Relationships

The Stark Law does provide an exception for bona fide employment relationships. This covers any amount paid by an employer to a physician (or an immediate family member of such physician) who has a bona fide employment relationship with the employer for the provision of services if:

1. The employment is for identifiable services;
2. The amount of the compensation:
   a. Is consistent with the fair market value of the services; and
   b. Is not determined in a manner that takes into account (directly or indirectly) the volume or value of any referrals by the referring physician.
3. The compensation is provided pursuant to an agreement that would be commercially reasonable even if no referrals were made to the employer.

Stark Exception for Personal Service Arrangements

A Stark exception also exists for personal service arrangements for situations that involve someone who is not a W-2 employee (e.g., medical director or on-call arrangements), if:

1. The arrangement is set out in writing, signed by the parties, and specifies the services covered by the arrangement;
2. The arrangement covers all the services to be provided by the physician (or an immediate family member of such physician) to the entity;
3. The aggregate services contracted for do not exceed those that are reasonable and necessary for the legitimate business purposes of the arrangement;
4. The term of the arrangement is for at least 1 year;
5. The compensation to be paid over the term of the arrangement is set in advance;
6. The compensation to be paid does not exceed fair market value;
7. The compensation to be paid is not determined in a manner that takes into account the volume or value of any referrals or other business generated between the parties; and
8. The services to be performed under the arrangement do not involve the counseling or promotion or a business arrangement or other activity that violates any state or federal law.

STARK LAW DEFINITION FOR FAIR MARKET VALUE

The definition of fair market value is very important under Stark. The term "fair market value" means the value in arm's-length transactions, consistent with the general market value. "General market value" means the price that an asset would bring as the result of bona fide bargaining between well-informed buyers and sellers who are not otherwise in a position to generate business for the other party, or the compensation that would be included in a service agreement as the result of bona fide bargaining between well-informed parties to the agreement who are not otherwise able to generate business for the other party, at the time of the service agreement.

Usually, the fair market price is the compensation that has been included in bona fide service agreements with comparable terms at the time of the agreement, where the compensation has not been determined in any manner that considers the volume or value of anticipated or actual referrals.

STARK LAW DEFINITION OF GROUP PRACTICE

As discussed further below, group practices may avail themselves of certain rules and exceptions regarding the allocation of overall profits and productivity bonuses. The term "group practice" means a group of two or more physicians legally organized as a partnership, professional corporation, foundation, not-for-profit corporation, faculty practice plan, or similar association:

1. In which each physician who is a member of the group provides substantially the full range of services the physician routinely provides, including medical care, consultation, diagnosis, or treatment, through the joint use of shared office space, facilities, equipment, and personnel;
2. For which substantially all the services of the physicians who are members of the group are provided through the group;
3. Are billed under a billing number assigned to the group and amounts so received are treated as receipts of the group;
4. In which the overhead expenses of and the income from the practice are distributed in accordance with methods previously determined;
5. In which no physician who is a member of the group directly or indirectly receives compensation based on the volume or value of referrals by the physician (with certain exceptions);
6. In which members of the group personally conduct no less than 75% of the physician-patient encounters of the group practice; and
7. Which meets such other standards as the Secretary may impose by regulation.

SPECIAL RULE FOR PROFIT SHARES AND PRODUCTIVITY BONUSES IN GROUP PRACTICES

A physician in a group practice may be paid a share of "overall profits" of the group, provided that the share is not determined in any manner that is directly related to the volume or value of referrals of DHS by the physician.

Additionally, a physician in the group practice may be paid a productivity bonus based on services that he or she has personally performed, or services "incident to" such personally performed services, or both, provided that the bonus is not determined in any manner that is directly related to the volume or value of referrals of DHS by the physician. Payments for services actually performed is probably the most often used method for these compensation arrangements.

"Overall profits" means 1) the group's entire profits derived from DHS payable by Medicare or Medicaid; or 2) the profits derived from DHS payable by

Medicare or Medicaid of any component of the group practice that consists of at least five physicians.

Overall profits should be divided in a reasonable and verifiable manner that is not directly related to the volume or value of the physician's referrals of DHS. The share of overall profits will be deemed not to relate directly to the volume or value of referrals if one of the following conditions is met:

1. The group's profits are divided *per capita* (for example, divided and allocated equally to each member of the group or per physician in the group); or
2. Revenues derived from DHS are distributed based on the distribution of the group practice's revenues attributed to services that are *not DHS* payable by any federal healthcare program or private payer; or
3. Revenues derived from DHS constitute *less than 5%* of the group practice's total revenues, and the allocated portion of those revenues to each physician in the group practice constitutes 5% or less of his or her total compensation from the group.

A *productivity bonus* must be calculated in a reasonable and verifiable manner that is not directly related to the volume or value of the physician's referrals of DHS. A productivity bonus will be deemed not to relate directly to the volume or value of referrals of DHS if one of the following conditions is met:

1. The bonus is based on the physician's *total patient encounters or RVUs*; or
2. The bonus is based on the allocation of the physician's compensation attributable to services that are *not DHS* payable by a federal healthcare program or private payer; or
3. Revenues derived from DHS are *less than 5%* of the group practice's total revenues, and the allocated portion of those revenues to each physician in the group practice constitutes 5% or less of his or her total compensation from the group practice.

Every medical group must maintain thorough documentation of the systems, calculations, and processes that are used to determine physician compensation.

SPECIAL RULES ON COMPENSATION

The following special rules apply for purposes of the Stark exceptions discussed above:

1. Compensation is considered "set in advance" if the aggregate compensation, a time-based or per-unit of service-based (whether per-use or per-service) amount, or a specific formula for calculating the compensation is set in an agreement between the parties *before* the furnishing of the items or services for which the compensation is to be paid. The formula for determining the compensation must be set forth in sufficient detail so that it can be objectively verified, and the formula may not be changed or modified during the course

of the agreement in any manner that takes into account the volume or value of referrals or other business generated by the referring physician. Since these agreements must have a duration of one year or more, in order to be set in advance, the compensation arrangements must be entered in writing prior to the beginning of each contract year.

2. Unit-based compensation (including time-based or per-unit of service-based compensation) is deemed not to consider "the volume or value of referrals" if the compensation is fair market value for services or items actually provided and does not vary during the course of the compensation arrangement in any manner that takes into account referrals of DHS.

   Unit-based compensation (including time-based or per-unit of service-based compensation) is deemed not to take into account "other business generated between the parties," provided that the compensation is fair market value for items and services actually provided and does not vary during the course of the compensation arrangement in any manner that takes into account referrals or other business generated by the referring physician, including private pay healthcare business. Note that services personally performed by the referring physician are not considered "other business generated" by the referring physician.

CONTRACTUALLY LIMITING REFERRALS

In certain circumstances, the Stark Law does allow a financial arrangement between a physician and a DHS entity to be conditioned on referrals to a specific entity. Specifically, a physician's compensation from a bona fide employer, within a clinically integrated network, under a managed care contract, or other contract for personal services may be conditioned on the physician's referrals to a particular provider, practitioner, or supplier, as long as the compensation arrangement meets all of the following conditions:

1. Is set in advance for the term of the agreement;

2. Is consistent with fair market value for services performed and the payment does not take into account the volume or value of anticipated or required referrals; and

3. Complies with both of the following conditions:

   a. The requirement to make referrals to a particular provider, practitioner, or supplier is set forth in a written agreement signed by the parties; and

   b. The requirement to make referrals to a particular provider, practitioner, or supplier does not apply if

      i. the patient expresses a preference for a different provider, practitioner, or supplier;

      ii. the patient's insurer determines the provider, practitioner, or supplier; or

      iii. the referral is not in the patient's best medical interests in the physician's judgment.

4. The required referrals relate solely to the physician's services covered by the scope of the employment or the contract, and the referral requirement is reasonably necessary to effectuate the legitimate business purposes of the compensation arrangement.

5. In no event may the physician be required to make referrals that relate to services that are not provided by the physician under the scope of his or her employment or contract.

THE ANTI-KICKBACK STATUTE

The anti-kickback statute (AKS) prohibits knowing or willful payments of any kind of inducement in return for referrals. Therefore, to avoid being attacked for a violation of the AKS, make sure that payments are not made with the intent to induce referrals or with the intent to limit medically necessary services for patients. Thankfully, safe harbors are available. Note that being outside of an AKS safe harbor does not mean that a compensation arrangement is illegal, but being within a safe harbor provides assurance that the arrangement will be free from attack. Being outside the safe harbor means that the parties will have to accept a certain degree of risk in the arrangement.

The most-used safe harbor is generally known as the "personal services and the management contracts" safe harbor. This requires that the physician compensation agreement meet seven standards:

1. The agreement must be in writing;
2. The agreement must describe all the services to be provided;
3. If the agreement is periodic, sporadic, or part-time, it must specify exactly the schedule of the intervals;
4. The agreement must be for not less than one year;
5. Compensation must be set in advance, consistent with fair market value, and not determined in a manner that takes into account the volume or value of referrals;
6. The arrangement cannot involve the counseling or promotion of a business that violates state or federal law and;
7. The aggregate services do not exceed those reasonable necessary to accomplish the commercially reasonable purposes of the agreement.

When parties enter these compensation agreements, determining what is set in advance, fair market value, and commercially reasonable, are the most difficult aspects of the agreements. Typically, it is necessary to engage a third-party valuation organization to review and comment upon the terms of the compensation agreement to ensure that the agreement meets these requirements. Generally, however, a good rule of thumb is that if the Stark exceptions are met, the compensation arrangement will also meet the anti-kickback safe harbor.

NOT-FOR-PROFIT TAX RULES

If a not-for-profit entity like a hospital is the employer, additional rules apply. It is illegal to allow "tax-exempt" dollars to be paid to "taxable" individual physicians unless the payment is justified by the delivery of services of equal value. Those services may only be compensated at fair market value. In these situations, fair market value should be determined by an independent third party or by comparison to an independent compensation survey. If private inurement or private benefit occurs, the hospital could lose its tax except status.

Once an RVU compensation system is established, the RVU structure must be reviewed by an independent third-party valuation consultant. Or, at the very least, it must be compared to a valuation survey to verify that the RVU system results in overall compensation that is competitive and within the ranges of compensation that is paid to other similar practitioners.

CREDENTIALING

It is worth noting that economic credentialing systems also can be linked to RVU compensation systems. Hospitals use economic credentialing to do physician profiling and loyalty determinations. To the extent that a physician scores poorly in their RVU compensation, a hospital that does economic credentialing can use the RVU statistics against a practitioner.

Economic credentialing has been challenged frequently in lawsuits. However, hospitals have successfully justified the practice in most cases in those states when the matter is not profitability by law.

THE MEDICARE ACCESS AND CHIP REAUTHORIZATION ACT (MACRA), MIPS, AND APMS

The most recent development with significant impact on physician compensation is the Medicare Access and CHIP Reauthorization Act (MACRA) enacted in 2015. MACRA changes the way Medicare pays for professional services provided by physicians and non-physician practitioners. Beginning in 2019, physicians will be paid under one of two tracks: the Merit-Based Incentive Payment System (MIPS) or under advanced alternative payment models (APMs). Medicare will continue to use the RVU-based fees established in the physician fee schedule to compensate physicians. However, the actual payments received by a physician will, in many cases, be adjusted to reflect penalties or bonuses earned by the physician under MIPS and APMs. The specific adjustment will be based on the track in which the physician participates.

Most physicians will be paid under the MIPS, which is the default payment track. Under MIPS, physicians will be evaluated based on their performance in four categories: quality, cost, practice improvement activities, and advancing care information, such as meaningful use of electronic health records (EHR).

Each physician will receive a score, which will be compared to a threshold score calculated annually by CMS. Physicians above the threshold score will receive a bonus payment and those below the threshold score will receive a negative adjustment. Physicians will be evaluated two years prior to applicable payments, which means that for 2019 payments, CMS will evaluate the physician's performance in 2017. The potential payment adjustments increase over time, from ±4% in 2019 to ±9% in 2021 and beyond.

In contrast, physicians who decide to participate in certain APMs will not be subject to MIPS requirements and payment adjustments; instead, qualifying physicians (known as "qualifying participants," or QPs) will receive a lump-sum bonus payment of 5% of their revenues paid under the physician fee schedule each year, from 2019 through 2024.

To become QPs, physicians must provide a certain, significant percentage of their services through a qualified advanced APM. To qualify as an advanced APM, a payment model must require use of a certified EHR, tie some amount of payment to quality metrics, and require providers to take on downside risk. In 2017, only certain Medicare payment models qualified, including Tracks 2 and 3 of the Medicare Shared Savings Program, the Next Generation Accountable Care Organization model, the Comprehensive Care for Joint Replacement bundled payment program, and the Comprehensive Primary Care Plus medical home model.

Beginning in 2019, physicians will also receive advanced APM credit for certain risk-bearing arrangements with non-fee-for-service Medicare payers, including Medicare Advantage plans, state Medicaid programs, and commercial plans.

DHS entities that contract with physicians will need to consider how the potential positive and negative payment adjustments will affect those contracts, particularly in light of fair market value as discussed above. Significantly, the MACRA does not include any waiver of the Stark or anti-kickback laws. Therefore, physician compensation arrangements that attempt to address or incorporate the MACRA payment adjustments will still need to comply with those laws, including any applicable exceptions or safe harbors.

SUMMARY

RVU compensation systems are a recognized lawful system for determining productivity bonuses. However, other legal requirements must be met to ensure that overall compensation is lawfully paid. It is best to make sure that compensation is fair market value, commercially reasonable, and set in advance in a written agreement of one year or more.

CHAPTER 6

The Playbook for wRVU-Based Alignment Structures and Alignment Models

Today, RVUs are the prevailing system for monitoring physician productivity and determining their allowable reimbursement. Medicare annually establishes a physician fee schedule based on current procedural terminology (CPT) codes to determine payment for more than 7,500 physician services. The payment for each service depends on the RVUs, ranked on a common scale to the resources used to provide each service, which ultimately becomes each code's RVU value.

A total RVU value is comprised of three components: the expenses of the physician's practice (PE RVU), the professional liability (malpractice) insurance component (MP RVU), and the overall physician work or professional component (wRVU). Although the actual percentages of each component differ across services, the approximate Medicare expenditures for the work, practice expense, and professional liability are 52%, 44%, and 4% of the total RVU value, respectively. The calculation Medicare uses to determine the value of the reimbursement entails multiplying a pre-determined and assigned dollar conversion factor by each RVU and is the same regardless of the specialty of the physician, establishing greater standardization. While it is adjusted for geographic differences in costs and other factors, RVUs still represent the greatest level of standardization for reimbursement and productivity (Coker Group, 2014).

Since their adoption, RVUs undeniably remain the most accurate methodology for interpreting operating results within the practice and, specifically, tracking and analyzing physician productivity. Very few metrics establish a truly consistent standard of measurement within the context of performance. Gross charges may be used as a standard because they are calculated prior to any adjustments for contractual allowances, bad debts, etc. However, there is no standard for where gross charges are set. They can be changed easily at the press of a button with any adjustments to the fee schedule the practice's decision. For example, if the practice increases its fee schedule, the total gross charges will increase, but the actual amount of collections may not increase commensurately.

Using gross charges to measure productivity can be misleading for both practice administrators and physicians, as it is unlikely that the true revenue realized has changed. Since their adoption into the medical world by CMS over 20 years ago, RVUs have remained the primary vehicle for productivity measurement in medical practice, and the CMS standard for reimbursement. Throughout their tenure, they have provided greater insights into the value of medical services that are performed and they inherently consider variances in the resources needed versus those consumed by providers when rendering professional services (Coker Group, 2014).

THE RELEVANCE OF PRODUCTIVITY UNITS

Using RVUs as the basis of productivity measurement aligns reimbursement and the perceived work effort of the physician with the government's expectations because CMS determines the value of all three RVU components based on current market conditions. CMS also considers recommendations from the Relative Value Scale Update Committee (RUC), which is a panel of physicians and medical advisors who make recommendations to CMS on the resources required to provide a medical service.

The Relative Value Scale Update Committee

The goal of the RUC is to represent the entire medical profession, with 21 of its 31 members appointed by medical specialty societies. The members must meet the following specifications:

1. The specialty is recognized by the American Board of Medical Specialties;
2. The members represent a specialty with a large percentage of physicians in patient care; and
3. The members represent a specialty with high percentages of Medicare expenditures.

The remaining members include four seats that rotate every two years (two internal medicine subspecialties, one primary care, and one for any other specialty), the RUC chair, the co-chair of the RUC Healthcare Professionals Advisory Committee Review Board, and representatives from the American Medical Association (AMA), American Osteopathic Association (AOA), the chair of the Practice Expense Review Committee, and CPT Editorial Panel. The AMA Board of Trustees selects the RUC chair and the AMA representative to the RUC, while the specialty societies nominate individual members of the RUC. The AMA must approve all members of the RUC (American Medical Association, 2017) .

While CMS ultimately makes the final decision on the value of each medical service, the RUC submits feedback annually on these values and whether they are appropriately accounting for the time spent (by both physician and staff) and the supplies and equipment involved to determine reimbursement. The RUC works closely with the medical specialty societies to review the current RVU values and determine if they appropriately value physician work effort and reimbursement. The RUC follows a step-by-step process to review new or revised codes each year (American Medical Association, 2017).

1. CPT Editorial Panel's new or revised codes, along with CMS and RUC-identified "misvalued" services are transmitted to the RUC staff.

2. Members of the RUC Advisory Committee and specialty society staff review the summary and indicate their societies' interest in developing a recommendation.

3. For those CPT codes requiring input, the respective medical societies are required to survey at least 30 practicing physicians, using a list of 10–20 services that have been selected by the specialty RVS committee, to ascertain the work involved.

4. The specialty RVS committees review the results and prepare their recommendations to the RUC. If multiple societies are involved in developing a recommendation, they are encouraged to develop and present a consensus recommendation to the RUC.

5. The specialty advisors present recommendations at the RUC meeting and defend their proposals.

6. The RUC may either adopt, refer back, or modify a specialty society's recommendation before submitting to CMS. A two-thirds majority is required for the final recommendation to CMS.

7. The RUC's recommendations are forwarded to CMS for their review.

8. The Medicare Physician Fee Schedule is published after CMS reviews all RUC recommendations.

Historically, the acceptance rate for the RUC's recommendations has been more than 90% each year, which demonstrates the significant impact and influence a single committee has over a metric that is responsible for compensating the majority of physicians practicing today. The RVU values are not only responsible for directly reimbursing physicians treating Medicare patients, as well as any other payer who uses the RBRVS as the underpinnings of their reimbursement methodology, but also play a role in determining compensation for any physician whose compensation plan utilizes a work RVU foundation. Thus, the RUC's influence extends well beyond their recommendations to CMS.

The Physician Work Component

For this discussion, we will continue to focus on the physician work component, also known as the wRVU. wRVUs are advantageous because they are payer-blind and their value is based on the actual work effort of the physician for a given service. Other measures of productivity, such as gross charges or net collections, are not an accurate reflection of the work effort a physician expends on a certain service because they are reliant on a practice's fee schedule or payer mix.

However, when using wRVUs as the basis for compensation, it is still imperative that the practice also factors net income into the overall economics to ensure a wRVU-based compensation mechanism is financially viable. Meaning, in a private practice setting, it is advantageous to use wRVUs as an unbiased measurement of physician work effort to allocate collections, income available for distribution, or other components of the compensation methodology. In this manner, physicians' compensation is subject to a more unbiased allocation methodology.

For example, if collections are the allocation methodology, payer mix can significantly impact the allocation. This is not the case with wRVUs. The approach to utilizing wRVUs differs from the employment setting where physicians are often compensated at a set rate per wRVU that is determined using industry market data to ensure a level of compensation that is considered fair market value.

However, it is important that the health system or hospital still align the overall economics of the physician compensation plan with their revenue sources. Regardless of the underlying data supporting the compensation plan, it must still be affordable.

With newer payment models becoming more common (e.g., medical homes, bundled payments, etc.), productivity and, by extension, wRVUs will continue to play a pivotal role in determining physician reimbursement. Regardless of the U.S. healthcare system moving into an era when value-based measures such as quality and patient outcomes factor into compensation structures, productivity-based payments (fee for service) will persist (Coker Group, 2014). wRVUs can be used to establish baseline work expectations for physicians and ensure there is a sustained balance between volume and quality.

Over the past 7–10 years, the U.S. healthcare system has slowly shifted from one that compensates solely on the number of procedures performed to one where physicians are required to meet a minimum quality standard. As the industry continues to shift, volume will remain important to prevent a complete shift to a system that focuses only on quality.

Although it may sound great on the surface, eliminating volume from the equation entirely could cause a number of issues, such as decreased revenue from lack of volume and decreased patient access due to physicians seeing fewer patients. However, a better balance between volume and quality will keep on moving the needle on improved healthcare in the U.S.

To use an extreme example, no physician will be successful seeing one patient a day, but doing it at an extremely high level of quality. There must be a reasonable level of volume, but it must be balanced with a high level of quality.

To this end and as an example of the changing landscape, the RUC focused on an initiative to address payment for non-face-to-face services for 20 minutes or more of clinical staff management time to address multiple significant chronic conditions during their recommendations for the 2015 Medicare physician fee schedule. As a result, a new CPT code (99490) was introduced in 2015 to reimburse for patient management (American Medical Association, 2017).

The Shift from Volume to Value

Government and commercial payers alike are continuing to base reimbursement on a fee-for-service platform while shifting the focus to quality through value-based measures and payment modifiers. The introduction of the Medicare Access and CHIP Reauthorization Act (MACRA) solidified this approach. MACRA, which passed in April 2015, replaced the sustainable growth rate (SGR) as a way for CMS to adjust payments to physicians to drive both quality and control costs within the Medicare system. Further, MACRA consolidated multiple quality reporting programs into the Merit-based Incentive Payment System (MIPS) and also provided incentives for participation in alternative payment models (APMs) and advanced alternative payment models (AAPMs).

MIPS measures participant performance through a composite score that takes into account four factors: quality, resource use, clinical practice improvement activities (CPIA), and advancing care information (ACI). MIPS consolidated these four previously voluntary performance measuring programs into one mandatory reporting system. Once fully implemented in 2019, the MIPS composite performance score (CPS) that factors in the scores from all four categories described above will be used to adjust physician payments up or down by 4% in the first year, increasing to an up or down adjustment of 9% in 2022.

A MIPS-eligible clinician's payment adjustment percentage is based on the relationship between his CPS and the MIPS performance threshold. Thus, MIPS is taking a fee-for-service platform and adjusting the payment based on the achievement of value-based measures, as was discussed in detail in Chapter 4 (Coker Group, 2016). Because MIPS is grounded in a fee-for-service methodology, wRVUs will remain as essential to the reimbursement paradigm as they provide the payment foundation for physician professional services. Therefore, as wRVUs will continue to play an important role in reimbursement, they should also continue to play an important role in physician compensation.

At least in the foreseeable future, wRVUs will provide the foundation for reimbursement and compensation alike, with fee-for-service payments adjusted based on the achievement of value-based metrics. Although other important measures of productivity and performance are being introduced, it is unlikely the wRVU component will ever disappear, as volume will continue to play a role as patient demand increases.

OTHER MEASURES OF PRODUCTIVITY

With the shift to value-based payments, other measures of physician productivity have been introduced, particularly in primary care where most of the changes have occurred. In 2007, the Institute for Healthcare Improvement (IHI) launched the Triple Aim initiative, which focused on three objectives: improving the patient experience of care, improving the health of populations, and reducing the per-capita cost of healthcare.

To achieve these goals, health systems, hospitals, and physicians had to shift their focus from acute, specialized episodes of care to a broader focus on primary and preventive care for a population of patients (McCarthy & Klein, 2010). One particular metric, panel size, is now being considered in concert with wRVU productivity to emphasize population health management. The wRVUs associated with this type of evaluation/management work are lower than the procedure heavy work of specialists, with the added burden of managing a patient's overall health and chronic conditions cost-effectively.

Payment for Panel Size

Some payers are beginning to tie a portion of primary care reimbursement to a physician's panel size to recognize the population health management component. Here, the physician is reimbursed at a set rate per member with the expectation that the physician will effectively manage the cost of healthcare for her panel of patients with the remainder of reimbursement still tied to fee for service. Thus, the shift to population health management more closely integrates volume with value in primary care specialties. Of course, capitation takes this much further by tying the totality of reimbursement to panel size.

The American Medical Group Association (AMGA), a widely used resource for physician compensation data throughout the healthcare industry, defines panel size as the count of unique patients a physician has seen in the past 18 months, which is a somewhat standard definition in the industry (AMGA, 2017). In this calculation, patients are automatically assigned to the physician if they have seen only that physician for all visits within the last three years. In cases where the patient has seen multiple physicians, an algorithm is needed to determine where to assign the patient, as the patient should be assigned to only a single provider. For example, the patient is assigned to the physician whom they saw most often, or, if the patient saw multiple physicians the same amount of times, they are assigned to the physician seen most recently.

Some challenges surrounding tracking and attributing patients to physicians are related mainly to how patients are utilizing primary care services. In some cases, patients see multiple physicians in an 18-month period simply because they saw the first available physician as opposed to seeing the same physician multiple times.

Also, patients often see advanced practice providers (APPs) as their primary care provider, and the treatment of APP panels differs in each organization. Some organizations assign patients to the APP whereas others assign patients to the supervising physician. If the APP is productive and functions independent of the supervising physician, as is often the case in primary care, the aggregate panel data will be skewed for the physician.

With the focus on panel size growing within primary care compensation models, it is important to consistently establish panel size to incentivize access and promote team-based care, and to recognize required work that is not wRVU-generating in managing a population of patients.

Often, panel size represents only 3–5% of total compensation and the panel incentive compensation pool is funded using wRVUs, again continuing to bring volume into the equation. A physician's wRVUs are weighted for the various components of compensation: wRVU productivity, panel size (for primary care), and quality. Then, the wRVUs are used to fund the compensation pools for each of the incentives.

In the case of panel size, the panel incentive pool is divided by the primary care total panel size to determine a per-member rate of compensation. The incentive can be used to reward increases in panel size past an established baseline or can be paid based simply on the respective panel size of each primary care provider, recognizing the care management that is required. In either case, the incentive is compensated at the per-member rate.

The panel incentive can also be integrated with the quality incentive. Instead of the physician receiving the full per-member payment based on respective panel size, this amount represents the physician's incentive opportunity which is then compensated based on the achievement of quality metrics. In this manner, improved quality of care and cost-saving measures directly linked to population health management will influence physician compensation and, ultimately, behavior.

Implementing panel size can, even in a small way, spark discussion on important topics such as patient attribution, acuity, population health management, etc. As discussed above, patient attribution can be tricky depending on how the patient is interacting with the organization and whether or not APPs are present in the practice. Before introducing a panel incentive, the practice must be able to track and assign patients to each physician and/or APP who is providing care consistently.

Another key consideration when implementing a panel incentive is patient acuity. It would be unreasonable to expect the same panel size from a physician managing all geriatric patients versus one managing all young healthy patients. Thus, it is important to find a method to adjust the panel size based on patient acuity. The simplest way to do this is to adjust by age, weighting patients who are older in years as heavier than those younger in years. Another alternative, albeit more complex and subject to available data, is weighting based on patient risk scores or some other metrics that take into consideration both the health and the age of the patient.

Many of the current primary care models that include panel size as an incentive keep these two components of productivity separate, with a large percentage of the compensation pool allocated to wRVU productivity and a small percentage of the pool allocated to panel size and other quality/non-productivity-based metrics. Following this methodology, there are two productivity components and one quality/non-productivity component of any compensation model. Another approach is to combine wRVU and panel productivity into one metric, which can be termed a work equivalent value unit (wEVU). The wEVU is a blend of panel size and wRVU productivity (see Figure 6.1). wRVUs and panel size can be weighted equally (for example, at 50%) to determine wEVUs. The total cash compensation (TCC) to wEVU ratio is determined by taking TCC market data for each specialty and dividing it by the median wEVU for such specialty. The weight of each component can be adjusted to adapt the model to the changing reimbursement environment annually. The panel size component establishes basic work expectations for full-time physicians, leads to more consistent performance amongst providers, and helps to manage future staffing and patient needs, while the wRVU component helps to focus on actually seeing the patients in the panel, and generating revenue in the fee-for-service arena.

Along with the evolving healthcare environment, there continues to be a greater focus on factors other than productivity within compensation models and reimbursement paradigms. A fundamental desire of many hospitals and practices is to build these incentives into the existing compensation mechanism such that the same measures will drive the reimbursement vehicle and the compensation vehicle. However, working to achieve balance when doing so is vital. As an example, if 90% of professional services revenue is tied to fee-for-service reimbursement, having a compensation mechanism that is tied to 90% of value-based reimbursement is not functional because it incentivizes different behaviors

FIGURE 6.1. Work Equivalent Value Unit (wEVU)–A Blend of Panel Size and wRVU Productivity

wEVU Analysis	Weight	National Market Data Percentiles - FTE Adjusted			
		25th %ile	50th %ile	75th %ile	90th %ile
Family Medicine					
wRVUs	50%	1,993.50	2,447.50	2,932.50	3,509.00
Panel	50%	716.75	919.50	1,197.50	1,447.06
wEVU		**2,710.25**	**3,367.00**	**4,130.00**	**4,956.06**
TCC per wEVU		*$52.56[1]*	*$62.95*	*$78.75*	*$101.43*
Internal Medicine					
wRVUs	50%	1,885.50	2,372.50	2,884.00	3,546.50
Panel	50%	706.50	918.00	1,186.50	1,427.53
wEVU		**2,592.00**	**3,290.50**	**4,070.50**	**4,974.03**
TCC per wEVU		*$56.22*	*$68.09*	*$85.57*	*$112.69*
Primary Care					
wRVUs	50%	1,939.50	2,410.00	2,908.25	3,527.75
Panel	50%	711.63	918.75	1,192.00	1,437.30
wEVU		**2,651.13**	**3,328.75**	**4,100.25**	**4,965.05**
TCC per wEVU		*$54.37*	*$65.49*	*$82.12*	*$107.00*

[1]$176,954 / 3,367

than those tied to reimbursement. Thus, it is important for an organization to design compensation methodologies using an *allocation-of-value* approach (see Figure 6.2) so they can easily adapt to the shift in focus of both the healthcare industry and payer contracts. This concept is unpacked further in Chapter 4.

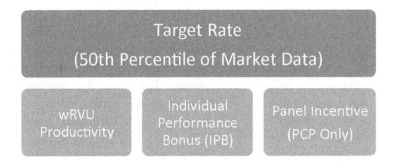

FIGURE 6.2. Allocation-of-Value Approach

Ultimately, the quality metrics implemented should align with the overall quality and cost-saving goals of the organization as well as metrics that impact fee-for-service reimbursement. It is more important to ensure that the metrics chosen are meaningful and can be accurately tracked. Many of the challenges surrounding implementing this type of incentive relate to an organization's ability to capture data and create meaningful reports. Once these systems are in place, other questions arise such as the accuracy of the underlying data, the objectivity of the established measures, the applicability of the measures to both the physician and the organization, and the ability to measure impact.

All these concerns are secondary, however, if the funds are not available to incentivize physicians. With this in mind, there needs to be a balance between the metrics chosen and the value assigned. In other words, $50,000 in value should not be tied to a single metric nor should $5,000 be tied to 20 metrics.

Time also has been used as a measurement of productivity. Time value units (TVU) are of greater significance and applicability in some settings. This measure is especially applicable and used as a system for the valuation of dental procedures and the development of dental fees—also called a relative time-cost unit (RTCU) system. However, this system also applies to medical practices for certain specialties where TVUs may be a fairer method of productivity and cost assessment than RVUs.

The application is just as it infers: instead of the traditional RVU measurement based upon the actual work and related cost of performing the professional services, the unit of productivity is based on the amount of time required to complete the work. This has a narrow application and is not as standardized as the RVU system. TVUs seem to have their greatest application in specialties such as in cardiology, where the time that is required to perform a particular function is a better methodology than the RVU system.

Many cardiology practices have developed a system similar to an RVU measurement of productivity, which applies TVUs based on the time required to complete each professional work product. For example, a cardiologist who is trained to read echocardiograms can do so within a relatively short period—perhaps as little as five minutes—whereas an encounter of a diagnostic nature directly with the patient will undoubtedly take much longer. In looking at RVU values, the value of reading the echocardiogram is far greater than the E/M code that would support the diagnostic encounter. This position could be argued from either point of view and the decision as to which standard is most appropriate ultimately should be that of the physicians and administrative leadership. In some practices, the utilization of both TVUs and RVUs is applied with a weighting of the two similar to the previously illustrated wEVU concept. In this case, time is the other factor instead of panel size.

CMS publishes a time study for all CPT codes billed in a given year with the average time spent on any given procedure. Organizations can develop TVUs using the average time reported per procedure as the baseline for these units. CMS typically posts updated time studies for the previous year by September. This information is also useful when attempting to divide or assess productivity for global payments.

FUTURE RELEVANCE OF RVUS

The introduction of value-based care and the integration of CMS's previously separate fee-for-service and fee-for-value reimbursement often calls into question the continued relevance of RVUs. Regardless of the continued shift of the healthcare industry to focus on quality and value, there will always be a need for an unbiased metric to measure a physician's work effort, especially with the CMS's continued push for bundled payments and the impact of capitation in certain markets. RVUs can still be a means to tabulate, aggregate, and measure performance in conjunction with the achievement of quality and cost-saving metrics. As value-based payments trend toward the *new normal*, new productivity measures likely will continue to be developed and, in our opinion, continue to incorporate or meld with RVUs to drive volume.

Bundled payments are rapidly becoming a common form of reimbursement for services in the American healthcare system. Fundamentally, bundled payments work by bundling together the payments for a single healthcare service (procedure or treatment of a clinical condition over a period of time), including the professional and technical payments for any single service. Providers who come together to deliver services under such arrangements are paid the bundled price, which they are expected to divide per pre-determined allocation methods as determined by the providers (Coker Group, 2017).

As an example, let's review the global payment for routine obstetrical (OB) services. We previously discussed a time study CMS publishes that outlines the average time per procedure as well as all associated E/M codes that support the procedure code. In the case of the OB global CPT codes, there are both pre- and post-natal visits, as well as the hospital stay, embedded in the global payment, which is billed at the time of delivery.

The global payment provides reimbursement for several facets in the continuum of OB care, and patients, more often than not, see multiple providers throughout a nine-month pregnancy. Thus, an impartial methodology such as a wRVU allocation is needed to appropriately compensate all of the providers for the work associated with the global payment for routine OB services. The organization can break down the global codes (59400, 59510) into components and assign the wRVUs for each piece to the physician or provider who performed the work to determine compensation for the OB care based on the work effort expended. Bundled payments take this concept one step further where the single payment for episodes of treatments are shared by both the hospital and the physician.

Capitated payments, also known simply as capitation, involve paying a healthcare organization a fixed payment per year/month per covered life and then asking the provider organization to meet all the needs of a broad patient population for that single payment. Popular during the 1980s and 1990s, this payment method was not found to change the cost trajectory significantly within the healthcare industry.

Capitation is usually used to pay for population health management services and puts providers at risk for overall spend, readmission rates, and length of stay (Coker Group, 2017). Capitation is fundamentally the opposite of fee for service in that each time the physician renders services to a patient, it results in a cost to the physician that otherwise would not have been incurred. Thus, the incentive in capitation is to limit or control the number of services rendered to patients to maximize profitability.

Similar to bundled and global payments, RVUs can come into play when tracking the cost expenditures of the physician, who is compensated at a set rate per member. Further, panel size is useful to track the total volume and acuity of the physician's assigned patients. The combination of these metrics determines the physician's allocation of the capitated payment (i.e., set payment per member), and the cost involved in managing the health of the physician's panel. Under a capitated model, it may make sense to derive base compensation from panel size by using a per-member-per-month (PMPM) amount multiplied by the physician's panel size. The PMPM amount is established using the *private practice* model (i.e., revenue minus expenses) such that physician compensation is representative of the net income available. A portion of the PMPM rate (approximately 85%) could be guaranteed as base compensation with the rest at risk based on the completion of performance metrics tied to cost-saving measures.

CONCLUSION

As we consider RVUs and related matters, it is safe to say that RVUs and derivatives thereof are here to stay. They are useful in measuring direct productivity of medical practice providers, and they are valuable in determining cost indicators such as staffing costs per RVU, total overhead per RVU, etc.

The introduction of MIPS establishes fee for service as the baseline of reimbursement for the foreseeable future, with measures for quality and cost-saving initiatives adjusting the fee-for-service payment rather than replacing it entirely. Finally, there will always be a need to value physician work effort that is unbiased (Coker Group, 2014).

REFERENCES

American Medical Association. (2017, August 17). *2017 RVS Update Process.* AMA. Retrieved from https://www.ama-assn.org/sites/default/files/media-browser/public/rbrvs/ruc-update-booklet_0.pdf

American Medical Association. (2017, August 17). An Introduction to the RUC. AMA. Retrieved from https://www.ama-assn.org/sites/default/files/media-browser/public/rbrvs/introduction-to-the-ruc-updated.pdf

American Medical Association. (2017, August 28). *Composition of the RVS Update Committee (RUC).* AMA. Retrieved from https://www.ama-assn.org/about-us/composition-rvs-update-committee-ruc

AMGA. (2017). *Survey Questionnaire and Specialty Definitions,* AMGA Medical Group Compensation and Productivity Survey AMGA. Retrieved from: http://www.physiciancompensation.org/PDFs/2017RJSPV/surveyQuestionnaire.pdf

Coker Group. (2014). *RVUs at Work.* Phoenix, MD: Greenbranch Publishing.

Coker Group. (2016). *MACRA: Redefining How CMS Pays Doctors.* MACRA Whitepaper. Alpharetta, GA; The Coker Group.

Coker Group. (2017, January 30). *Bundled Payments: What Are the Essentials You Need to Know?* Bundled Payments Whitepaper. Alpharetta, GA: The Coker Group.

McCarthy, D., & Klein, S. (2010, July 22). *The Triple Aim Journey: Improving Population Health and Patients' Experience of Care, While Reducing Costs.* The Commonwealth Fund. Retrieved from http://www.commonwealthfund.org/publications/case-studies/2010/jul/triple-aim-improving-population-health

CHAPTER 7

Value Units and Technology

While the concept of using RVUs as a performance measurement tool is nothing new, the technology being leveraged around these metrics has vastly improved and goes far beyond RVU data compiled on a spreadsheet. Historically, the technology needed and used for RVU tracking and strategies was managed by pulling data retrospectively from a medical billing system. This data was then exported to a Microsoft Excel spreadsheet or manually reentered.

The data was not dynamic and after producing was often considered meaningless given the fluid nature of any medical practice. Additionally, the data was almost exclusively used as a tool for determining physician compensation and for keeping compensation equitable among providers. It also helped with reducing any imbalances in reimbursement.

In theory, RVUs are all equal, so a provider has the same incentive to see someone with insurance versus a patient without coverage. As reimbursement models shift from volume to value, the RVU system is now being looked at to monitor quality and outcome. Further, it is even showing up as a metric for developing strategies such as mergers and acquisitions.

One significant gap in the RVU system is that not all procedures are associated with a value unit without the support of a modifier. Modifiers are unique codes added to CPT codes to describe variances in a procedure. This area is one where providers have benefited significantly from technology by programming their systems to alert them when modifiers are needed based on their exam notes and orders. However, this technology is not without its critics. Some argue these notices coach or influence a provider to use higher codes, a practice commonly called "upcoding." Others consider it to be a helpful reminder tool, much like a warning light to change the oil in a car.

There is also the concern of over-trusting a system to make these decisions for the provider. Many assume if something is computer generated it must be correct, which is not always the case. By engineering (programming) a system as a "default-driven" template, electronic health records (EHRs) can assign codes and produce boilerplate words that may not accurately reflect the physicians' treatment of the patient. A provider can come to rely on the wisdom of his or her system too heavily and allow it to take over in decision making if not careful. The Centers for Medicare and Medicaid Services (CMS) makes it explicitly clear the provider is ultimately responsible for his coding, even when assisted by an EHR or a staff member who is a scribe.

Another aspect of leveraging IT to assist with RVU monitoring and reporting is vendor accountability and commitment. Many practices and hospitals purchase software with defects and have no pathways for remediating these problems. In fact, most vendors' contracts explicitly exclude any responsibility for system defects and any liability in the event of incorrect coding. The contract may even specifically state that the software is NOT a substitution for provider coding, despite the fact it is promoted to assist with coding and charge capture. Vendors should be required to be accountable for defects, including any fines or penalties caused by their software. While the provider is ultimately responsible, the vendor MUST be held as accountable also.

Figure 7.1 provides an excerpt from an actual vendor contract excluding itself from any liability related to system and provider coding.

9.4   Disclaimer of Warranties; Databases; Content Third Party Software. ▇▇▇▇▇shall not be liable for any specific settings or databases embedded within the Programs. ▇▇▇▇▇ does not warrant the accuracy of codes, prices, Content, or other data contained in the Programs or any third party software incorporated into the Programs. Information reflecting prices is not a quotation or offer to sell or purchase. The clinical information contained in the Programs, including that contained in the Content, or any third party software incorporated into the Programs is intended as a supplement to, and not a substitute for, the knowledge, expertise, skill, and judgment of physicians, pharmacists, or other healthcare professionals in patient care. The absence of a warning for a given drug or drug combination shall not be construed to indicate that the drug or drug combination is safe, appropriate, or effective in any given patient. Billing codes, including without limitation ICD and CPT codes, which might be suggested by the Program are merely suggestions based upon the amount of documentation completed, and such codes are not intended to be a substitute for the healthcare professional's judgment. Customer is responsible for ensuring that billing codes entered into the Content are appropriate for the level of documentation completed. Any hard copy documents or images that are scanned and saved as files within the Program, and any digital images imported as files into the Program, are to be used for documentation purposes only and not for diagnostic purposes. ▇▇▇▇▇ shall not be liable for the content, accuracy, clarity, or resolution of any scanned images or digital images.

FIGURE 7.1. Sample Vendor Contract Disclaimer

Another common area where RVUs and IT intersect is during projects involving IT adoption and its impact on provider productivity. RVU tracking can be a useful tool to evaluate the impact of automation, especially provider productivity during the adoption of EHRs. Many organizations use RVUs as a historical benchmark to determine if an EHR is having an undesirable impact on productivity. In some cases, an organization may even agree to compensate its providers using the RVU average before the adoption of an EHR for a period. This provision allows the providers to deliberately slow down their patient volume during their training period without any adverse financial consequences. Also, it relieves the pressure of trying to see a full patient load while adjusting to a new computer system.

Tracking RVUs during and after an IT project can also be helpful in determining if there has been any increase in performance resulting from automation and modernization. It can also help to drill down on specific issues, such as coding and charge capture. The careful monitoring of RVUs should occur after any major IT projects in which charge capturing and clinical documentation are involved.

Finally, the latest trend in managing RVUs from an IT perspective is the concept of leveraging analytics and data performance dashboards. We know that one of the most common uses of RVUs is to compare physicians, peer-to-peer, by specialty within the practice or by using external industry benchmark data. However, with advanced data analytics, we can dive deeper and explore some important RVU ratios. These ratios can be obtained by combining RVU results with other practice variables, such as costs, which can produce an average cost per RVU ratio or payments to produce average payments per RVU.

In our research for this chapter, we enlisted input from Jose Valero, who is a data analytics expert and software developer of a vendor diagnostic tool called DashboardMD, which enables the use of data within existing IT system. Once the data is extracted, it is displayed in an easy-to-read dashboard that can be pointed specifically at various key performance indicators based on the preference of the leadership or data steward (see Figure 7.2). We asked Mr. Valero for some specific examples of how advanced data analytics could be combined with RVUs to provide enhanced reports. Here were just a few examples:

- ***RVUs per Work Day = Total RVUs/Number of Days Worked***

Look at calculating average wRVUs per work day for each provider. It's a consistent and daily measure of productivity that is not affected by providers taking time off or holidays.

This metric trended over time paints a much better picture of a provider's quality time seeing patients.

First, you'll need to produce a count for actual work days. This information can be attained by counting dates of service during the calculation period. Then, take the total RVUs and divide by the number of work days to obtain an average number of wRVUs per work day. You can calculate this metric per provider, facility, or practice.

When trended over time, this simple ratio may tell you if a provider is indeed working more or less over time. Better still, when trended against patient visit counts, this measure may show if a provider's coding levels have increased or decreased. That may be an indication that the provider is seeing more or less complex patients.

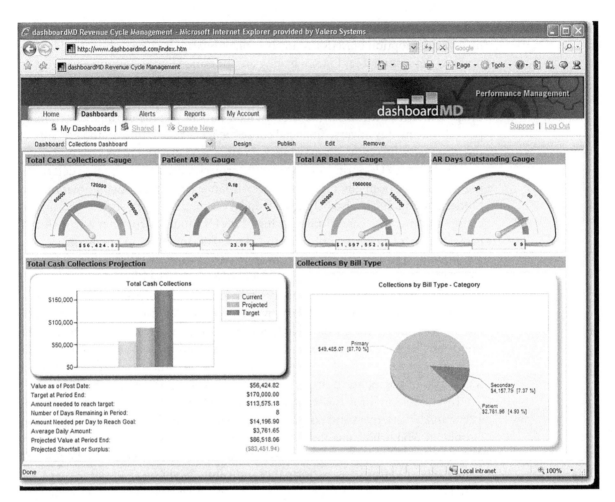

FIGURE 7.2. DashboardMD

- *RVUs per Visit = Total RVUs / Total Visits*

Another way to get a better sense of whether a provider is seeing more patients or seeing patients that may be more complex, take the total number of RVUs and divide by the total number of visits to produce average RVUs per visit.

- *RVUs per Patient = Total RVUs / Number of Unique Patients Seen*

To isolate the complexity per patient a bit further, take the total RVUs and divide them by the number of unique patients seen to produce a ratio of RVUs per patient.

- *Payments per RVU*

Payments per RVU or payments per wRVU could be considered the best of the bunch. It cuts through all the fog of fee schedules, collection, and adjustment rates. It's just good old dollars deposited per resource or work unit. The formula is simple enough: divide total payments RVU or by wRVU.

Calculate total payments and total wRVU values for each of your top payers and look at what contracts may be most profitable. Divide the total payments by the total wRVUs for each payer, and you'll get an amount per wRVU value per payer. This is essentially the number of dollars you are getting paid by that payer for each RVU work unit. Notice the variations of each contract. If the work efforts are equal across the board, you might consider that the plans that pay you the most per RVU work unit are the most profitable.

- *Cost per RVU and Provider Cost per wRVU*

Here's one that everyone can quickly put together. Divide the total practice costs for a year by your total RVUs across the board and you'll come up with practice cost per RVU. It's a great number to have in your back pocket when analyzing plans and comparing payments per RVU.

To calculate the cost per wRVU accurately, tally up only the provider compensation costs for the year. Otherwise, the numbers will be way off the mark.

- *Calculated Gross Profit per RVU = Payments per RVU – Cost per RVU*

Now that you've calculated payments per RVU and cost per RVU, go ahead and subtract to attain a calculated gross profit per RVU. This number can tell you about how many dollars you make per RVU.

You can take it a step further and calculate it separately for each of your top payers using payer-specific values for payments per RVU.

- *wRVU E/M Acuity Ratio*

RVUs also can be used to track coding compliance variance over time or compare among physicians. By taking your total wRVU values for all E/M visits and dividing the result by the number of units for those E/M visits, you get an average wRVU value for all E/M visits rolled up. We call this the wRVU acuity ratio.

This value is used to compare the coding levels quickly across physicians by specialty. The higher the acuity ratio, the higher the overall coding is. Conversely, the lower the acuity ratio, the lower the overall coding.

The calculation is a simple ratio of work RVU values per unit billed for each service code group.

Look at the example calculations for a batch of established office visits under the outpatient services charted in Figure 7.3.

FIGURE 7.3. Outpatient Services Chart			
CPT Code	wRVU	Units	Total wRVU (Units * wRVU Value)
99211	0.18	5	0.90
99212	0.48	30	14.40
99213	0.97	100	97.00
99214	1.50	20	30.00
99215	2.11	5	10.55
TOTALS		160	152.85

wRVU Acuity Ratio = Total wRVU / Units
152.85 / 160 = 0.96

Interestingly, the wRVU value for 99213 is 0.97. So, in this example, we can conclude that the provider is billing at about the same work acuity level as a Level 3 visit or a 99213.

The following are common definitions for many of the RVU abbreviations and formulas frequently used in RVU calculations and/or when performing an analysis. We also include links to additional resources that are updated frequently.

- *Formulas, Definitions, and Resources*

  wRVU = The work component

  peRVU = The practice expense component

  mpRVU = The malpractice expense component

  GPCI = Geographic Pricing Cost Index. Commonly pronounced "Gypsy"

  CF = Medicare Conversion Factor = $35.99 for CY 2018

  MA = Modifier Adjustments

  Medicare Allowable Payments= Total RVUs * Conversion Factor

  Total RVU= [(wRVUs * Work GPCI) +

  (peRVUs * Practice Expense GPCI) +

  (mpRVUs * Malpractice GPCI)]

  Total RVU = CPT Code Total RVU Value * MA

- *RVU Ratios*

  Average RVU per Visit = Total RVUs / Total Visits

  Average RVUs per Work Day = Total RVUs / Days Worked

  Practice Cost per RVU = Total RVUs / Total Practice Cost

  Provider Cost per wRVU = Total wRVUs / Total Provider Compensation

  Payments per wRVU = Total wRVU / Total Payments

  wRVU E&M Acuity Ratio = Total wRVU for E&M Visits / E&M Visits

- *RVU Values on CMS.GOV*

  https://www.cms.gov/Medicare/Medicare-Fee-for-Service-Payment/PhysicianFeeSched/PFS-Relative-Value-Files.html

- *Reference Notes*
  - Make sure to include only fully adjudicated charges and try to use a full year's worth of data. The more data, the better but six months should be considered a minimum if a full year's worth is not available.
  - Reporting or calculation period can be any specified time range such as a month, quarter, or year.
  - When calculating ratios, be sure to combine values from the same reporting period.
  - Note that visits are unique encounters and patient counts are unique patients.
  - A simple method for trending is to calculate a series of monthly numbers or monthly averages and compare three or more.

CHAPTER 8

Management in a Hybrid Reimbursement Environment Performance Measurement

Work relative value units (wRVUs) are here to stay. As a practical measure, they've been established as a fairly consistent measurement tool relative to physician productivity for many years.

The comforting aspect about wRVUs is that they provide, and have provided, a relatively stable litmus for "production" since deployment in the late 1980s through the early 1990s. As the broader healthcare market moves closer toward value-based care and reimbursement, wRVUs will serve as a valuable measurement tool relative to both provider production and care quality, in terms of measurement and outcomes.

A nuance to utilizing wRVUs in production and quality measurement is both agreement and buy-in from providers. Providers must first concur that these measures will offer no biases to the system and will help providers hold each other accountable for their work. This acceptance can be the most challenging aspect of utilizing wRVUs in performance and production measurement. Crucial to deployment for performance is the use of a physician-partner and leader who can assist the management (i.e., *non-clinical team*) in herding the cats to ensure compliance and relevancy of wRVUs as a measurement tool.

Lastly, using wRVUs as a measure of production and performance does not artificially incentivize providers to offer and/or provide unnecessary care. Instead, they simply measure the work being performed and can aid management in reviewing staffing levels (both provider and clinic/management), time commitment (e.g., to a satellite office), and expenses

wRVUs can be a useful tool among many to offer sound, objective standards by which providers can measure and monitor a variety of business aspects.

ANALYTICS APPLICATION

For far too long, healthcare managers in both employed physician networks (EPNs) and private medical practices have failed to harness the valuable data available to them within their practices. Whether in clinical care management or practice administration/management, administrators and clinicians have been remiss to utilize the data at their fingertips.

Historically, aggregation and management of data in healthcare have been woefully lacking. This deficit is not necessarily due to administrative inertia but instead, in some instances, to deficient legacy reporting capabilities and the multitude of disparate information technology (IT) components that don't *talk* (e.g., EMR, digital imaging, labs, etc.). However, over the last 10–15 years, those reporting structures and the opportunity to mine data have improved exponentially.

This *data dearth* is an interesting dichotomy because of the acuity of the "business" of healthcare—of helping people toward better health. Widget makers understand and manage their data better than people in healthcare, whether it's inventory management, cost/pricing data, or quality and outcomes data.

With that said, more tools are available to better harness and manage data and enable systems to "talk" with one another to share data, such as analytics tools for value-based care delivery, data warehousing, and image-sharing technologies.

wRVUs can be a valuable tool in business management. While providers may voice consternation that wRVUs don't necessarily measure the "real work" they perform, the RVU construct has existed since the early 1990s. wRVUs, for the good or the bad, have evolved into the accepted standard measure of "work" performed by providers over the course of time. And, aside from home-grown one-offs, such as wRVU-like measures built by practices to monitor work or reward, wRVUs have been the most consistent tool available to managers and administrators. Compensation plans also have been built utilizing wRVUs as a component piece for years.

Because of the relative standardization of wRVUs, using them to perform analytics is fairly straightforward. Every year, Medicare publishes the wRVUs assigned to each CPT code. It is easy to obtain the Medicare Part B Physician Fee Schedule from the CMS website. The data can then be download and exported via Excel spreadsheet. Once the data is downloaded, administrators can run their provider's billed CPT frequency and multiply the output by the wRVUs assigned to each CPT code.

Figure 8.1 displays the frequency of established patients seen by Dr. X and also the cumulative wRVUs that he generated by treating those patients. (wRVU values for this example are fictional.)

CPT	Frequency	wRVU Value	Total wRVUs
99211	1	0.75	0.75
99212	5	0.95	4.75
99213	10	1.05	10.5
99214	6	1.3	7.8
99215	3	1.5	4.5
Total:	25		28.3

FIGURE 8.1. Dr X wRVUs Generated

Dr. X has a fairly standard Gaussian distribution of his established visit codes. As indicated, the wRVU value per CPT code increases as the code level increases because there is more work involved in seeing patients with a greater level of severity.

In summary, Dr. X has generated 28.3 wRVUs by seeing established patients. This calculation can be performed for each billing provider within a group and each CPT code billed.

The reader should know that what you bill is not what you get paid, but it is worth noting that what you billed does carry with it a work value that needs to be accounted for in terms of productivity measures.

Figure 8.2 shows a practice that generated $10M in net revenue (before expenses—cash in the door) recently. The providers in this group (all physicians) generated 75,000 wRVUs. The practice collected $133.33 per wRVU generated during 2016.

2016 Revenue
$ 10,000,000
wRVUs
75,000
Rev/wRVU
$ 133.33

FIGURE 8.2. Practice Revenue in 2016

As an aside, if the practice's expenses are $150/wRVU, there is a darker underlying issue.

The data illustrated in Figure 8.2 should be readily available in practice management reporting systems. Often, though, per-wRVU collections rates are not calculated so some manual work must be performed.

On the whole, what we've displayed in Figure 8.2 does not paint an entire picture. Is $10M in revenue good? Are 75,000 wRVUs performed good? If we collect $133.33 per wRVU, are we generating large margins or just covering costs?

Figure 8.3 gives us more insight, at least into production and revenue.

Figure 8.3 provides a look at data for a 10-physician medical practice. Flowing from the left-hand column to the right, it gives us insight into each physician's productivity for 2017. As seen, a total of 75,000 wRVUs were produced. Note that in the column *Budgeted wRVUs,* our target for 2017 was 75,470 so the practice fell short by 470 wRVUs or 1%. At $133.33/wRVU collections, our budgeted revenues would have fallen short by approximately $63,000 (470 wRVUs x $133.33).

The underlying question is "is 75,000 wRVUs a good number?" As we review the 2016 data, we see that the practice produced 71,000 wRVUs in 2016, so they

Analytics Dashboard - YTD 1/1/2016 - 12/31/2016

	2017 wRVUs	Budgeted wRVUs	wRVUs vs Budgeted	% Change	Last Year 2016 wRVUs	wRVUs CYTD v PYTD	CYTD vs PYTD % Change	Collections/ wRVU
Dr. 1	4,500	5,870	(1,370)	-23%	5,600	-1100	-20%	$ 155
Dr. 2	10,000	9,000	1,000	11%	9,900	100	1%	$ 129
Dr. 3	5,000	5,100	(100)	-2%	4,500	500	11%	$ 105
Dr. 4	2,200	4,000	(1,800)	-45%	3,000	-800	-27%	$ 125
Dr. 5	8,800	9,000	(200)	-2%	8,500	300	4%	$ 155
Dr. 6	5,000	5,000	-	0%	4,500	500	11%	$ 118
Dr. 7	15,000	12,500	2,500	20%	11,000	4000	36%	$ 115
Dr. 8	12,500	12,000	500	4%	11,000	1500	14%	$ 140
Dr. 9	10,000	9,000	1,000	11%	9,500	500	5%	$ 145
Dr. 10	2,000	4,000	(2,000)	-50%	3,500	-1500	-43%	$ 165
Total:	75,000	75,470	(470)	-1%	71,000	4000	6%	

FIGURE 8.3. Analytics Dashboard

realized a 6% gain or 4,000 wRVUs which should, all things being equal, translate into more than $500,000 in additional revenue.

Lastly, we see that while the practice has generated $133.33/wRVU, a vast disparity exists in collections/wRVU by physician—an issue worthy of investigation.

In Figure 8.4 three columns are added to the right side of the dashboard.

Analytics Dashboard - YTD 1/1/2016 - 12/31/2016

	2017 wRVUs	Budgeted wRVUs	wRVUs vs Budgeted	% Change	Last Year 2016 wRVUs	wRVUs CYTD v PYTD	CYTD vs PYTD % Change	Collections/ wRVU	Expenses per wRVU	Margin per wRVU	Margin %
Dr. 1	4,500	5,870	(1,370)	-23%	5,600	-1100	-20%	$ 155	$ 90	$ 65	42%
Dr. 2	10,000	9,000	1,000	11%	9,900	100	1%	$ 129	$ 90	$ 39	30%
Dr. 3	5,000	5,100	(100)	-2%	4,500	500	11%	$ 105	$ 100	$ 5	5%
Dr. 4	2,200	4,000	(1,800)	-45%	3,000	-800	-27%	$ 125	$ 100	$ 25	20%
Dr. 5	8,800	9,000	(200)	-2%	8,500	300	4%	$ 155	$ 100	$ 55	35%
Dr. 6	5,000	5,000	-	0%	4,500	500	11%	$ 118	$ 90	$ 28	24%
Dr. 7	15,000	12,500	2,500	20%	11,000	4000	36%	$ 115	$ 90	$ 25	22%
Dr. 8	12,500	12,000	500	4%	11,000	1500	14%	$ 140	$ 90	$ 50	36%
Dr. 9	10,000	9,000	1,000	11%	9,500	500	5%	$ 145	$ 100	$ 45	31%
Dr. 10	2,000	4,000	(2,000)	-50%	3,500	-1500	-43%	$ 165	$ 100	$ 65	39%
Total:	75,000	75,470	(470)	-1%	71,000	4000	6%				

FIGURE 8.4. Analytics Dashboard

The dashboard suggests that the fictional group has a cost structure that varies by provider; some providers have $90/wRVU in expenses attributed to them while others are charged $100/wRVU in expenses. (Perhaps they are liable for a share of both direct and indirect costs.)

This piece of the analysis better explains the *value* of our revenue and the impact of expenses. That is, examining both the expense and revenue sides of the ledger enables us to have a better understanding of the financial well-being of the practice and, at this level of analytics, empowers us to examine and opine on problem areas vis-à-vis financial performance. Additionally, this high-level analysis will point the management team toward areas requiring further investigation.

As noted in Figure 8.4, the additional columns added indicate the profitability by provider in the practice. The dashboard also offers a look at the margin and margin percent that the providers are generating. In this example, the profit margin in the practice ranges from 5% to 42%.

It is difficult to examine these figures and see a common thread. For instance, one might contemplate that a $100/wRVU expense allocation would render lower margins. However, in Figure 8.4, some of the greatest margins derive from those providers with $100/wRVU cost allocations.

Pushing the math further, the practice runs about $7M in expenses (based on current wRVU output and allocated expenditures per wRVU), which means that the practice has an overhead ratio of approximately 70%. Stated differently, the practice pays .70 cents of every dollar earned on expenses. In a vacuum, this seems like a high overhead rate. However, if only three providers are shareholders, they may split the remaining $3M as a partner distribution.

The dashboard in Figure 8.4 defines for the practice physicians whose practice structure and style, apropos of expenses, may require further analysis and review.

ACCOUNTABILITY

Non-clinical managers, working with their provider-advocate(s), need established measures to both monitor and measure outcomes. They also need a strong associate leader in the operations arena. The leadership could be a physician/administrator management dyad team (supported by a nimble Board or Executive Committee that is subordinate to the Board). The task is to operationalize and deploy the strategic plan while simultaneously holding both clinicians and other staff members accountable to the greater mission.

Figure 8.5 denotes a management structure in which the administrator is paired with a managing partner to administer the operational aspects of the business. In this example, the Board parses out defined roles to an Executive Committee to handle operational aspects of the practice.

This form of *dyad management* empowers and enables administrators to perform their jobs and utilize their physician lead to address performance issues, peer-to-peer. Asking a non-clinician to manage difficult situations with physicians can be tenuous. That said, the physician lead should be a strong personality who *understands* practice operations and is an honest broker when difficult situations arise. This structure is essential because it empowers the lead provider to engage his or her peers and offers management arm's-length dealings with the provider on issues that can be fairly sensitive.

Again, wRVUs are not the sole nor ultimate measurement tool for "work", but they are the current gold standard and a measurement tool for the practice. Thus, by using a dashboard similar to Figure 8.4, we can begin to use RVUs to help manage the practice objectively. (Utilization requires transparency in data,

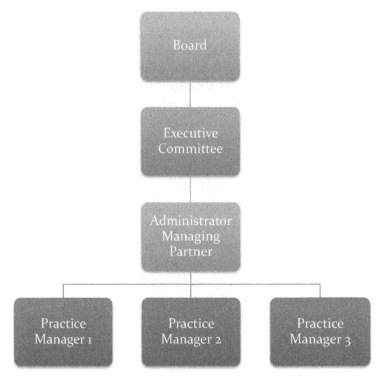

FIGURE 8.5. Management Structure Sample

veracity of data, and physician-shareholder [or leadership] willingness to embrace the tool.)

Once deployed, wRVUs can help us budget where we are relative to expectations. The administrator and shareholders (leadership) can establish provider wRVU production expectations and, as noted in Figure 8.1, utilize the average $/wRVU revenue collection to budget net revenue expectations per provider. Additionally, for administrators who acutely understand their expense logic and are able to apply expenses/wRVUs by provider, it enables the management team to carefully analyze cost components by provider as well as margin and profitability.

For example, the data provided in Figure 8.4 should lead the practice to areas that are important to review. For example, Dr. 1 finished the year 23% below his budgeted wRVUs, which we know, based on revenue/wRVU, means a revenue shortfall of nearly $200,000 relative to budgeted wRVUs. The practice should wonder why Dr. 1 is so much lower than both budgeted wRVUs but also to the prior year's wRVU production (2016's data indicates production of 5,600 wRVUs). It should be noted that during the year, Dr. 1 collected at $155/ wRVU–significantly higher than most of his peers–had an expense structure of $90/wRVU and generated a 42% profit margin. Of course, those numbers would be significantly better if Dr. 1 met his budgeted wRVUs for 2017.

In this simple example, there are myriad opportunities to drill down into the data and embrace the wRVU structure, empowering the administrator and his or her physician (or senior leader) to manage the practice objectively and hold the providers accountable for their production, spend, and margins. Also, the revenue/wRVU disparity may lead management to both question and investigate the revenue cycle of the practice.

Of course, nothing occurs in a vacuum and, as such, our data as presented in Figure 8.4 requires a deeper dive into the what and why of the current results. Maybe Dr. 3 provides a sub-specialty service that the practice deems necessary to the service area and leadership has concluded that a 5% margin is satisfactory.

As discussed, to utilize wRVUs in both a dashboard and as an accountability tool, physician buy-in is essential. A component of that buy-in includes specific education regarding wRVUs, their history, and baselining. The reasoning behind deployment should be explained to practitioners.

Once acceptance and buy-in are obtained, ample time should be apportioned for lead up to deployment. A 3- to 6-month window will offer providers peace with the data and enable them to understand the starting point of the exercise. Also, real data can be deployed, in draft form, to offer a snapshot of where the practice currently resides. While this exercise may be uncomfortable, it will offer clarity, an aspect crucial to effective management of a medical operation.

An wRVU dashboard should be deployed at the beginning of a calendar year to keep accounting clean. It certainly can be implemented in a rolling or partial year, but many practices run calendar/fiscal year January 1–December 31.

Ideally, data should be reviewed monthly but at least quarterly to keep shareholders and/or leadership fully engaged. (If wRVUs are utilized in compensation plans, a monthly review may be warranted.) wRVU goals can be established annually relative to revenue and expenses, strategic planning, etc. This requires a micro-understanding of the areas the provider practices, such as patient demand, geopolitics, socioeconomic demands locally and regionally, etc.

The interesting aspect and maybe finer point about utilizing wRVUs in accountability measures is that it removes the need to perform complicated analytics throughout the practice. If all providers/shareholders agree on the methodology, the mathematics behind wRVU "accounting" is fairly simple.

Lastly, this model may be used to assist with clinical outcomes and *value* of the same. Understanding the cost/wRVU in a value-based environment may be a crucial component in ensuring that expenses are managed and sound margins are maintained in a bundled payment or value-based reimbursement scheme.

STRATEGIC PLANNING

Note: The *strategic planning* aspect of this chapter is a discussion about how wRVUs can be brought to bear in the strategic planning process.

Strategic planning is not one-dimensional. It is (or should be) the conscious effort of a multi-variable process defining major goals that an organization strives to achieve over the course of a set period. It is, decidedly, iterative. Inherent in that calculus, of course, is the "value" of business expansion (or contraction) and its impact on finances and operations.

While the strategic plan is a guiding roadmap to business operations, for the purposes of this chapter, we'll assume that strategic planning includes a careful analysis of component pieces that an organization determines are essential to either growing or shrinking operations in a given area. That is, the strategic plan will include the overarching system approach to operational penetration in geographic areas that make sense (e.g., under-served areas, telemedicine programs in outlying regions, etc.) and will include an analysis of suggested changes to current operational structure and footprint of the overall practice.

The strategic planning process should include a pro forma that addresses items contemplated in the plan, such as capital expenditures (*capex*), staffing, office expansion, service line expansion, and IT.

The plan should include the diagnosis and current standing of the business with a concerted and candid review of its strengths and weaknesses. This analysis applies to both EPNs and private practices.

When performed properly, the strategic planning dynamic involves multiple variables, including geopolitics, current patient volumes, strength (or lack thereof) of the health system in place, available (and reasonably priced) real estate, and a thoughtful and objective analysis of the business's strengths, weaknesses, opportunities, and threats (SWOT) and vision and mission.

A SWOT analysis is an honest examination of where the business is relative to its stated goals: Can it get to the *next level*? Does it have the human resources to start a new office? What is the competition in that space currently doing?

Let's presume the sample practice discussed earlier wants to expand to another locale. The non-exhaustive list of component pieces in the strategic planning process should include reviewing current demographics of the patients who reside in that area because, theoretically, many of them will now seek care in the new office location. A zip code analysis should be run pairing the patients with the wRVUs generated on each patient who may not seek care at the "old" office location.

The planning should account for a certain level of *cannibalization* or out-migration of current patients. Also, thought should be given to possible expansion and referral sources in the region and a marketing plan should be generated and budgeted. Other costs included in the pro forma consist of budgeted items (new staff/shared staff), build-out costs, IT needs, marketing needs and ramp up, payer component (e.g., contracts extend to the new region/area?), and expected production.

The practice may go as far as understanding revenue based on wRVUs. For instance, by understanding the collected revenues for a year or two, the practice can break down the collections per wRVU generated. As an aside, if the practice has a compensation plan that incorporates a wRVU component, this may actually be a worthwhile exercise in that the practice can evaluate the pay per wRVU with the collections per wRVU to determine if they are paying out more than they receive in revenue.

Develop a business plan that includes the pro forma for the component pieces mentioned above.

An argument can rightfully be made that using wRVUs to budget out financial expectations can be dangerous. However, we suggest that other avenues of budgeting in terms of expansion can be equally as precarious. In Figure 8.6, we have culled out both Drs. 1 and 7.

Provider	2017 wRVUs	Collections	Collections/ wRVU	Comp	Comp/ wRVU	Expenses /wRVU
Dr. 1	4,500	$ 697,500	$ 155	$ 400,000	$ 89	$ 90
Dr. 7	15,000	$ 1,725,000	$ 115	$ 500,000	$ 33	$ 90

FIGURE 8.6. Pro forma Example

In this practice, the physicians are not on a wRVU compensation model, but the administrator does examine compensation relative to wRVU production. As shown, Dr. 1 has a $90 expense/wRVU ratio but is compensated $89/wRVU. And, our margin examination earlier in the chapter was pure expense, not physician salaries. So, perhaps Dr. 1 is a partner in the practice and will receive some of the $3M (30% overall margin) remaining after year's end.

However, Dr. 7 is much more productive and, while he earns more in compensation relative to Dr. 1, his comp/wRVU is relatively low and he has $90/wRVU in expenses. Utilizing Dr. 7 in the new market may make sense, owing to exigencies and other variables. She is highly productive and a relatively low drag on expenses.

Our sample practice (Figures 8.1–8.3) seeks to expand into Market X. They have performed all of the requisite strategic planning initiatives and have done thorough research to determine that the choice, at least subjectively, appears to be the right choice. However, the practice lead, with his physician counterpart, must ensure that the math makes sense, that the financials will stand up to the rigors of the additional operation.

Given all of the inputs and variables, the practice has determined that the overview in Figure 8.7 is a fair representation of the expected financial performance in Market X over the next three years.

Strategic Plan Production Estimate		
Year 1	Year 2	Year 3
12,000	30,000	38,000
Main Office wRVU Loss*		
5,500	5,500	5,500
New Revenue		
$ 866,667	$ 3,266,667	$ 4,333,333
Projected Expenses		
$ (625,000)	$ (450,000)	$ (450,000)
Projected Net Revenue		
$ 241,667	$ 2,816,667	$ 3,883,333

*Patients are lost "once" in year 1

FIGURE 8.7. Strategic Plan Production Estimate

As indicated in Figure 8.7, in year 1, the practice expects 12,000 wRVUs to be produced at the new location. (Of course, all of the data driving this analysis rolls up into this easily digestible dashboard.) In presenting the data to the shareholders, it may be prudent to discount revenues or offer a range to be conservative. Also, it may be advisable to offer a range for expenses. (Unseen and/or unanticipated expenses generally throw a wrench in the veracity of profit and loss projections.)

In the analysis, the practice examined patient draw and geography and determined that the Main office will lose X number of patients that generated 5,000 wRVUs. They expect that almost all of these patients will visit the new office in Market X because it's convenient and their preferred physician will be there.

Utilizing the current revenue/wRVU ($133.33/wRVU), we extrapolate that the 12,000 wRVUs less the 5,000 wRVUs for out-migration will generate about $867K in revenue. They expect that the new office, in year 1, will cost the practice $625K, yielding approximately $242K in net revenue.

As seen in Years 2 and 3, margins are expected to grow significantly as the one-time, startup expenses wane and the office gains local market traction and growth via enhanced marketing out-referral outreach. Also note, in the analysis, the practice *lost* the 5,000 wRVUs in year 1 and those are static losses for Years 2 and 3. That is, those patients are gone *one time* and the practice carries that loss from its overall production figures. An argument can be made that the 12,000 wRVUs should be accounted for in Market X, and this is an internal practice discussion. However, this exercise shows the *net gain* to the *practice* in adding an office (e.g., the shift of patients from location Main to Market X).

Understand that this modeling is facile and very optimistic; the devil is in the details. Each line item assumption and consideration in Figure 8.6 is (should be) substantiated by a line item break down of all components related to both start up and ongoing operations. And, of course, the caveat is that the billing/collections remain static (e.g., $133.33/wRVU) and the production numbers and expense expectations are accurate. The takeaway should be the value, and use, of wRVUs in projecting out a strategy.

TACTICAL CONSIDERATIONS

The strategic plan must be boiled down to its tactical considerations to understand how micro-components of the larger scheme interplay. Once that occurs, operational/tactical aspects are front and center.

As noted previously, both the cost and revenue aspects of the profit and loss can be reviewed via wRVUs. Tactically, and broadly, we can deploy wRVUs to "realize" revenue and allocate costs. Harkening to both Figures 8.1 and 8.6, we can break down the tactical aspects of the strategy, combined in Figure 8.8.

The administrator of the practice is able to secure the same reimbursements in Market X as he has in location Main. So, all things being equal and assuming similar collection rates, the administrator budgets $133.33/wRVU for Market X.

His calculus regarding production is based on a progressive/incremental rollout of a provider presence in Market X. Tactically, it has been determined, and

	Strategic Plan Production Estimate		
	Year 1	Year 2	Year 3
	12,000	30,000	38,000
	Main Office wRVU Loss*		
2016	5,500	5,500	5,500
Revenue	New Revenue		
$ 10,000,000	$ 866,667	$ 3,266,667	$ 4,333,333
wRVUs	Projected Expenses		
75,000	$ (625,000)	$ (450,000)	$ (450,000)
Rev/wRVU	Projected Net Revenue		
$ 133.33	$ 241,667	$ 2,816,667	$ 3,883,333

wRVUs and Revenue

FIGURE 8.8. Strategic Plan Production Estimate

signed off by the Board, that Market X will have one FTE provider on site for three days per week. Also, the office will be open 10 hours per day to accommodate both "early risers" and patients who cannot be scheduled during working hours.

The administrator looks at three-days-per-week scheduling, for 10 hours per day, and doing the math, indicates that in Market X, the practice should generate 12,000 wRVUs in year one. The administrator then deducts the patients who arc not organic to the practice but who will now seek care in Market X rather than traveling to Main for care. While the 12,000 wRVUs are a true indication of work in Market X, the administrator is accommodating the loss of those patients at Main because there certainly will be reduced wRVUs in Main. (The administrator may wish to review the small impact of Market X on the overall business and parse out organic growth vs. a shifting of established patients from Main to Market X.)

The administrator then multiplies the 7,000 net wRVUs by the expected collection rate of $133.33 to determine expected revenue. At this point, for safety's sake, the administrator may wish to discount the expected revenues and/or offer administration a range of expected revenues in the off (but likely) chance that the practice does not perform to par, that patients don't migrate, that some patients leave, that some referrals are not realized.

The administrator has broken down the costs of year one. Those include added (though minimal) full-time staffing to ensure continuity and a full-time market presence, a reasonable rental rate in the new location (including a moderate build-out to accommodate the needs of the specialty), an IT backbone, marketing, etc.

As noted earlier, the physicians ranged between $90 to $100/wRVU in expenses. Since Market X is new, the administrator must determine which physicians will support Market X and/or use their per/wRVU expenses allocations (and other variables) or price out actual expenses for Market X. The unsavory aspect of using actual expenses is that if the practice is generally run on per/wRVU expense numbers, we enter a zone of multiple reporting structures that removes continuity. That said, the administrator can certainly run numbers based on both wRVUs and actual expenditures to align the two and determine disparities on an annual basis.

The tactical considerations roll into the overall strategic plan and should be managed by the operational dyad referenced earlier.

CONCLUSION

wRVUs are certainly not the only avenue by which to measure production, work, and revenue. However, over the last 20-plus years, they've become the standard as valuable, and fairly static, tools by which to measure, monitor, and impact medical practice operations. Given their nature, they can be deployed readily to analyze data, accountability, production, and revenue, and used as accountability tools in both strategic and tactical settings.

Use of wRVUs as a hard and fast measurement tool is predicated on team *buy-in*; that is, both the providers (clinicians) and non-providers must embrace their use as measurement tools.

wRVUs, as a reporting dashboard (or a portion of one), are powerful management tools that remove emotion and subjectivity from operations and clearly have value relative in benchmarking and analysis of provider production.

CHAPTER 9

Care Coordination Processes

The overarching imperative in the healthcare industry today is to improve quality of care and cost efficiency simultaneously. Unfortunately, the U. S. healthcare system ranks far behind other economically developed countries in both of these parameters. To improve outcomes and lower expenses, then, the system must be re-tooled to be more coordinated and efficient at the front lines of care delivery.

This chapter describes how care delivery at the exam room, operating room, bedside, home, and even virtual levels must be designed to function more effectively and efficiently. It also ties together the use of productivity-based work units (wRVUs) to these newer, more novel care delivery processes. Further, it explains how wRVUs can remain relevant in compensation plan design as the methods of delivering healthcare services continue to evolve.

We will begin by describing a method of care process design. The Care Process Design System provides a systematic approach to the creation of highly reliable and cost-effective workflows in the healthcare industry. Next, we will review the inexorable move of reimbursements from a volume-based to a more value-based model and how care coordination can improve the value delivered to the consumers of healthcare services.

We will also describe how management of clinical and financial operations in the healthcare system increasingly must be combined to provide optimal services to patients and populations. Finally, we will return to the discussion of wRVUs and their utility in measuring units of work in a more highly coordinated care system.

CARE PROCESS DESIGN

Care delivery in the healthcare system involves myriad processes and procedures that occur thousands of times a day across thousands of types of healthcare facilities. Whether you are talking about hospitals, physician practices, ambulatory surgery centers, imaging centers, rehabilitation facilities, nursing homes, hospice, or home care, the front-line delivery of care in each of these locations can be broken down into what is known as the care process unit or CPU. CPUs must have a well-defined start and stop point and usually involve individual or small teams of caregivers. Examples of CPUs include a visit for a diabetic patient in a primary care physician's office, a surgical procedure (such as total joint replacement) in a hospital's OR or outpatient surgery center, a physical therapy rehab session for a patient who has just undergone total joint replacement in a skilled nursing facility (SNF), and a home visit for post-operative wound care by a home health nurse.

The CPU then becomes the basic unit around which care process design is performed. Unfortunately, in the current system, many of these CPUs are not well-designed and function in a poorly coordinated ineffective and inefficient fashion. The purposeful design of the CPU through simple process mapping to understand the major steps in each CPU and application of evidence-based, best-practices to each step in the CPU can dramatically improve the quality and efficiency of these processes and procedures.

One of the guiding principles that should be used in this design process is to try and create better coordination of care within each CPU and across the clinical care continuum as CPUs are combined to create what are known as integrated practice units or IPUs. IPUs usually involve the coordinated care of a common clinical condition, such as diabetes mellitus or congestive heart failure, across the pre-acute, acute, and post-acute care environment. Improving the way in which care is delivered via IPUs has been shown in many cases to produce higher value (defined as quality per unit of cost) for the patients suffering from each of these conditions and the many other chronic illnesses that now plague our aging society.

Care coordination then involves the design of CPUs that integrate with others to form IPUs that are highly effective and efficient. Let's look at an example of how this might work for a patient with congestive heart failure:

The patient is a 66-year-old male with a history of several heart attacks. These acute events have weakened his heart to the point that he now suffers from chronic shortness of breath, swelling in the lower extremities, and exercise intolerance to the point of near immobility. He still lives at home where he is visited by a heart failure care coordinator three times a week. He communicates with the heart failure coordinator more frequently through a mobile app on his smartphone. The care coordinator also communicates, as needed, with the patient's heart failure specialist cardiologist on an as-needed basis.

The patient himself is seen once a month in the heart failure clinic by the cardiologist and her team of caregivers (nurse practitioners, medical assistants, EKG and echo techs, etc.). Since being under the coordinated care of this heart failure team, the patient has not required acute care hospitalization and has enjoyed improvements such as far less bothersome symptoms and more time at home to enjoy his family and hobbies. Before being enrolled in this coordinated heart failure care program, the patient required acute care in the hospital on a frequent basis (3-4 times per year) and was nearly incapacitated by his illness. His healthcare costs after enrollment in the program have also dropped precipitously given that he is requiring less expensive acute care and taking a more streamlined, inexpensive medication regimen than before when his medication list seemed to change with every provider visit.

This patient is enjoying the benefits of a well-designed and highly coordinated care process (IPU) that involves several sub-components (CPUs). These components include the home visits by the care coordinator; the use of a mobile app for education, monitoring, and communication; the heart failure clinic visits; and the care processes delivered in the clinic by the multi-disciplinary team members.

It should be noted, however, that the type of coordinated care described above does not happen frequently in the current healthcare system. Instead, care tends to be delivered via islands of providers (physicians, advanced practice providers, nurses, ancillary service providers, etc.) who infrequently communicate with each other and follows their own isolated processes and procedures. There is no coordination of care across the continuum and the disjointed care that is delivered results in poor-quality outcomes and extremely high costs.

Also to note is that one of the reasons care in the current system is so fragmented and disjointed is that the basic way care is reimbursed today primarily utilizes a fee-for-service model where there are no incentives for care coordination, improved quality, or cost control.

The recent introduction of value-based reimbursement models, such as the Medicare Access and CHIP Reauthorization Act (MACRA) should improve this situation and introduce incentives into the system that reward care coordination and other practices that enhance value (quality and cost) for the healthcare consumer.

VALUE-BASED UNITS AND CARE COORDINATION

Value-based care delivery as called for in the MACRA quality payment programs (QPP) will be measured via performance metrics such as the physician quality reporting system (PQRS) quality metrics and costs of care as reflected in claims data.

Care coordination, however, will be measured by attestation of MACRA participants as to how they have implemented care process improvement activities (CPIA) and utilized electronic health records (EHR) in advancing care information (ACI) to patients cared for under the MACRA quality payment programs.

CPIAs include 92 separate activities that can be broken down into six categories:

1. Care Coordination
2. Participation in an APM, including a Medical Home Model
3. Integrated Behavioral and Mental Health
4. Population Management
5. Patient Safety and Practice Assessment
6. Achieving Health Equity
7. Beneficiary Engagement
8. Expanded Practice Access
9. Emergency Preparedness and Response

All of these categories involve activities that are geared toward improving care processes and procedures to move the system from the disjointed, fragmented system we have today toward a more coordinated, safe, high-quality, low-cost, and patient-centered care delivery model.

The activities that providers must attest to doing via EHRs in the ACI category of MACRA include the following:

1. Performing a Security Risk Analysis
2. E-Prescribing
3. Providing Patient Access
4. Sending a Summary of Care
5. Requesting/Accepting a Summary of Care

Additional performance score measures include:

1. Providing Patient-Specific Education
2. Allowing for the Viewing, Downloading, and Transmission of Information in Coordination of Care through Patient Engagement
3. Providing Secure Messaging
4. Providing Patient-Generated Health Data
5. Reconciling Clinical Information
6. Reporting to an Immunization Registry or Other Data Registry Reporting

Finally, bonus scores can be achieved in the MACRA ACI category for:

1. Syndromic Surveillance Reporting
2. Specialized Registry Reporting
3. Electronic Case Reporting
4. Public Health Registry Reporting
5. Clinical Data Registry Reporting

So, here again, care coordination through the use of EHRs will be a big goal of this largest of all value-based reimbursement programs, once it is fully implemented in 2019.

Finally, as described for the quality and cost measures of MACRA in Chapter 2, it will be incumbent on employers and other providers to align wRVU compensation models with this reimbursement model and its various measures of performance. No longer will measures of volume production via wRVUs adequately serve as the full measure of a provider's work and performance. Instead, wRVUs will need to be combined with newer measures of performance, including those geared toward improvements in coordination of care to adequately measure and incentivize a provider's activities.

MANAGEMENT OF EFFICIENCY AND CARE COORDINATION

The role of the healthcare manager in a highly coordinated care model will be dramatically different than that which exists today in the volume-oriented operations most prevalent throughout the system.

Coordinated care management will require processes and procedures to follow evidence-based guidelines and to be choreographed in a way that eliminates waste and inefficiency. This will require managers to expand their lists of key performance indicators (KPIs) beyond such items as patient or procedural volumes, throughput, revenue generation, and expense accounting at the organizational, departmental, or unit level. They must begin to look at new KPIs such as adherence to best practice guidelines (e.g., number of eligible patients in a pediatric practice who received all of their necessary vaccines), true clinical outcomes (e.g., the mortality rates for seriously ill patients with conditions like pneumonia, heart failure, heart attack, or stroke), costs across the spectrum of care for a clinical condition (e.g., diabetes, renal failure or organ transplantation), and survey results that gauge the level of satisfaction with the experience of receiving or delivering care within a more coordinated care environment.

Further, one of the most important managerial roles in a high-value healthcare delivery system will be to eliminate non-value-added costs (which must first be identified through much more accurate cost accounting systems than those currently used in most healthcare organizations) without affecting quality outcomes and patient safety. This responsibility may, in fact, be best delegated to managers with both clinical and financial training who can best assess the data in both spheres and most particularly change clinical practices by eliminating unnecessary costs without affecting clinical quality.

REVENUE CYCLE FUNCTIONS IN CARE COORDINATION

As emphasized above, highly coordinated care delivery will require well-designed and managed care processes and procedures. Likewise, billing and collecting for these high-value services will also require new approaches and techniques.

The very beginning of the revenue cycle in a value-based, well-coordinated delivery system begins at the point of care. Here, clinical care providers will be required to document in the inpatient or outpatient medical record information that can then result in accurate diagnostic codes (ICD-10), diagnostic groupings (DRGs, APCs), procedure codes (CPT 4), and risk-adjustment factors (HCC and RAF). Furthermore, the clinical documentation must reflect the medical necessity of the care rendered for third-party payers to approve payment for services.

Making sure the front-end revenue cycle activities referenced earlier are done properly will require teams of experts and add to the complexity of revenue cycle management in healthcare organizations. Those organizations that ignore these steps in the revenue cycle, however, will put themselves in considerable jeopardy, both financially and legally. Identifying and eliminating fraud and abuse from the healthcare system is a high priority for many payers, especially the Centers for Medicaid and Medicare Services (CMS). Providers who don't demand that the initial steps in the revenue cycle process are done in compliance with all legal and regulatory requirements, do so at their own peril.

At the back-end of the revenue cycle (billing and collecting), the processes in a high-value, coordinated care environment will also become more complex. No longer will a simple invoice for services rendered and vigorous pursuit of payments suffice in this regard. Instead, accurate payments for coordinated care services will require submission of information regarding procedures, diagnoses, quality performance measures, hierarchical clinical conditions, and other risk-adjustment factors, along with clinical documentation of medical necessity to the payer.

Many services in a coordinated care environment will be bundled, adding more complexity to the process. For instance, all services related to an episode of care will be reimbursed via a single payment. While bundled payments have been shown to promote care coordination between providers, they will also demand tighter coordination between providers within the revenue cycle including the billing and collection process. This, in fact, has led many providers to band together into organizations, such as clinically integrated networks and accountable care organizations where coordinated care guidelines can be more easily developed and reimbursements more equitably and accurately distributed to the various providers of care.

As an example, consider a group of orthopedic surgeons, anesthesiologists, and rehab providers who come together with a hospital to contract on a bundled payment basis for total joint replacement surgery. Most bundled payment models involve payment on a fee-for-service basis to each of the above providers for services delivered along the coordinated care process (IPU) related to total joint surgery. Also, the providers are usually paid a bonus at the end of the episode of care for meeting certain quality metrics and providing services within a pre-determined budget. These shared savings and quality incentives must then be distributed to each of the participants in the bundle in a fair and equitable manner. This involves development of an income distribution model that all involved agree to up front so that timely and accurate distributions of revenue can be made once the care is delivered.

THE ROLE OF RVUS IN CARE COORDINATION

As providers attempt to design a more coordinated, value-based delivery system, RVUs will likely remain an important way in which services delivered in such a system are measured. While other measures of care quality and efficiency will likely be used alongside wRVUs in provider compensation models, it is unlikely that these measures will replace wRVUs anytime soon. This is because while performance measures will become more important, productivity measures will not cease to be an important element of consideration when determining how to pay providers.

In fact, productivity measures (wRVUs) are likely to become even more important in a value-based delivery system where care coordination is emphasized. This has to do with the fact that the aging of the population, the increased prevalence of chronic disease and healthcare reforms that have expanded access to health insurance coverage will increase demand for healthcare services, regardless of the reimbursement model.

The exception to the above may be in primary care, where providers in these specialties—general internal medicine, family practice, and general pediatrics—will become more engaged in population health management (PHM) and less concerned with care of individual patients. This may lead to the substitution of panel size (i.e., the number of patients in a population being managed by a primary care provider) for wRVUs in compensation models. PHM, however, will probably not be a major concern for medical or surgical specialists, and these providers will likely continue to have their productivity measured via wRVUs.

CONCLUSION

High-value, coordinated care delivery will require a significant change in not only the way healthcare services are reimbursed, but also changes in the way healthcare is delivered at the front lines of care. Managers and providers of healthcare services would be well-advised to study how the shift from volume to value within the healthcare system will affect their day-to-day activities and add to the challenges they regularly face.

It cannot be overstated how much change is occurring within the healthcare system. That said, the use of RVUs will remain relevant to measuring productivity and useful in determining compensation for volume production within an industry that will always need to concern itself with important aspects of healthcare delivery, such as access and throughput.

Indeed, the term *volume to value* may be somewhat of a misnomer, as value will likely never replace volume as an important element of the healthcare system, and providers will always need to attend to both volume and value to succeed.

CHAPTER 10

Conclusion and Summary Concerning Value Units

The question of whether relative value units (RVUs) will continue to be a significant performance measurement tool for physician and other provider practices is a valid one. As the industry appears to move (though slowly) in the direction of compensation models other than fee-for-volume reimbursement, the measurements of performance in RVUs is a legitimate concern. Given the information included in previous chapters, we can conclude that RVUs will continue to be a significant part of the performance evaluation for physicians and other ambulatory practice evaluation processes. The emphasis on value-based reimbursement, notwithstanding MACRA requirements (see Chapter 2), is not yet significant. Further, with the uncertainties of healthcare regulations in the United States (vis-à-vis, the Affordable Care Act and its existence going forward), the importance of productivity in RVUs will endure.

While one could argue that value-based reimbursement should entirely negate the importance of RVUs, we disagree. First, RVUs continue to create a standard relative to industry performance of comparing one provider to another. The benchmarks established that are based mainly on RVUs will remain valuable as we measure one provider against another. Next, we believe RVUs will continue to undergo refinement as (and if) value-based reimbursement grows and develops. We have examined certain caveats and alternatives to the standard RVU derivation processes to support this premise. Enhancements will carry on if and when value-based reimbursement becomes more pronounced.

Thus, the future of RVUs is reasonably stable and, while somewhat cloudy, is reasonably reliable.

NEW FORMS OF VALUE UNITS

As the industry evolves, new value units will rise to the surface, and the question of obsolescence of RVUs will quickly pale in significance. Over the years, other forms of value-based RVUs with some differing definitions have come forth and are in use in many settings today. As addressed in earlier chapters, we can conclude that the *playbook* for RVUs will endure—whether as *time value units*, *quality units*, or some combination thereof (along with standard productivity-based units).

One of the most compelling reasons for utilizing RVUs in the measurement and evaluation of provider performance in an ambulatory setting is that they are easy to understand. Thus, their application in management and performance monitoring is respected. Moreover, basing provider compensation on some level of such performance is effective.

Moving to varied forms of RVU measurement (i.e., not necessarily being confined to fee-for-volume productivity) might dilute the effectiveness of utilizing them as a management and evaluation tool. However, educating providers, helping them to acclimate to a hybrid form of RVU aggregation will mitigate this issue. RVUs, while based (at least in part) on something other than straight productivity (i.e., volume) will not only extend their applicability and usefulness, but will likely reestablish their prominence as the single best way to evaluate performance. (Note: We admit to our bias that RVUs, historically, are the most viable method for evaluating the performance of a professional provider generating professional fees in a practice or other medical/healthcare setting.)

The education process of this new "slant" on RVU aggregation must ensue as value-based reimbursement continues to develop. Clearly, MACRA and related units of measurement (see Chapter 2) will continue to underscore this premise. We can conclude the following: *RVUs will continue to have and fulfill a major role in the performance evaluation of providers. However, the formulation of RVUs (vis-à-vis, their history as being strictly volume-based) will likely change to add elements of quality and cost-savings metrics.*

STRATEGIC PLANNING IN THE NEW REIMBURSEMENT PARADIGM

Another area that warrants serious consideration in the context of RVUs is how to plan strategically around RVU evaluation in the new reimbursement structure. Most practice strategic planning does not (yet) consider value-based reimbursement as a major component of the overall payment/receipt processes. Despite MACRA and its importance and relevance, the private payers have yet to rise to the initially anticipated level of significance.

Will this happen in the future, and should strategic planning accommodate such considerations? The answers to those two questions are complicated at best as none of us have the proverbial crystal ball. However, strategic planning should consider value-based reimbursement, at least as to how they will affect RVUs. Most strategic planning today should contemplate traditional forms of reimbursement and, therefore, utilize RVUs traditionally.

Nonetheless, strategic planning initiatives should consider potential changes to the reimbursement paradigm to include more value-based metrics. Introduction and education of providers on those changes should begin.

As the government continues to push MACRA and its related MIPS and/or APMs, it will be interesting to see the resultant changes in RVU derivation. Few, if any, changes have occurred to date. It is difficult to speak to providers who are currently focused on providing excellent care to their patients and "making a decent living" to discuss any mechanisms other than the traditional productivity-based metrics. Therefore, chapters that address value-based units and related issues may seem too progressive and futuristic. Nonetheless, we must continue to stress that MACRA is "real." Its tenets tie to something other than volume-based reimbursement. Further, private payers tend to follow government programs in their design and overall requirements.

The reality of MACRA stresses the likelihood that private insurers will be getting on board with value-based reimbursement. This movement warrants the inclusion of value-based reimbursement in strategic planning.

CLINICAL INTEGRATION

Clinical integration has been an evolving concept over the past two decades. Our discussions here have covered elements of clinical integration and structure, particularly clinically integrated networks formed largely to respond to value-based reimbursement. Additionally, we have attempted to "connect the dots" between clinical integration, value-based reimbursement, and some changes in unit measurements (vis-à-vis, RVUs).

The jury is still out as to how elements of clinical integration will be applied in a more pervasive sense in our reimbursement structure. And in turn, how clinical integration will affect RVUs. In Chapter 8, we consider hybrid reimbursement environment structures and how best to consider them. We consider the difficulties all managers of practices face as to the relevance of these applications to the successful medical practice and related healthcare entity.

Moreover, in Chapter 10, we consider care coordination processes and how these are at the core of value-based reimbursement considerations. As such, the role of RVUs and care coordination, while somewhat nebulous, should continue to be pursued in preparation for changes.

CONCLUSIONS

We trust that the issues discussed in this book are not viewed as too "futuristic," as they are based on a balance of current and pragmatic practice operations while considering the changes that are on the immediate horizon. Regardless, we hope we have heightened the awareness among providers and managers of healthcare entities in that RVUs (volume- and value-based) will continue to be both relevant and instrumental in the future. There are many things to consider, and there are many unknown factors. As the horizon becomes the current landscape, we will know more and can react accordingly.

CPSIA information can be obtained
at www.ICGtesting.com
Printed in the USA
BVHW01s1802130718
521139BV00001B/1/P